Gout diet ar

A guide on gout natural remedies, home remedies, diet, treatment, prevention, recipes and current research.

by

Gilbert Goldstein

Published by: IMB publishing 2015

Table Of Contents

Chapter 1: Introduction To Gout

1. What Is Gout?

According to a study conducted by the National Institute of Arthritis and Musculoskeletal and Skin Diseases (NIAMS), around 6 million adults at the ages of 20 years or older have been diagnosed with gout. This shows how common this disease is, and it is more common in men, especially when they reach the age of 40 or above. However, women can also become susceptible to the disease after they reach menopause. Gout is one of the many forms of arthritis and is quite painful. The condition is caused when the amount of uric acid increases within the body. This excess uric acid is then converted into crystals by the body, which then accumulate within the joints, thereby causing pain. The starting point of this pain is usually the big toe. However, gout can also travel into other joints such as those of the knees, feet, elbows, wrists, ankles, and fingers.

2. Is Gout Serious?

While gout can be extremely painful, the condition is treatable with the right medications, treatment, and lifestyle. If you have recurring gout attacks that you do not take seriously or treat, then these attacks can eventually lead to damage in the joints. In some people, the uric acid crystals can even damage the kidneys by forming kidney stones. In other instances, these crystals can form tophi, a condition where bumps are formed underneath the skin. While tophi can be painless and harmless, they can sometimes form in positions and places that are awkward, for instance at the fingertips. In some cases, this tophi can become infected as well.

3. How Common Is The Occurrence Of Gout?

Gout is mostly known to affect more men compared to women, and the disease affects 1 in 200 adult individuals. In most cases, the first gout attack will happen when an individual reaches middle age. However, in other instances, younger people can also be affected by or develop the disease. Doctors often check family history for the disease because the disease tends to run in some families. In about 1 out of 5 cases of gout there will be a family history related to the disease. Your genetic makeup that you end up inheriting from your family plays a highly important role in determining whether you will be impacted by the disease or not.

4. Types Of Gout

Acute Gout

Acute gout is a type of gout where one or more of the joints gets affected, usually the big toe. The attacks can start at night and can be triggered with the usage of alcohol, having surgery, trauma, heart attack, having a diet rich in purine, and certain types of medications. The joints that are affected can swell up, be extremely tender, and turn red. The early attacks of gout can, in most cases, subside after the initial 3 to 10 days. Some peeling of the skin from the region of the joint that has been affected may also arise. If proper treatment is not received, then the attacks can even last for a longer duration of time. More than 50% of the acute gout attack sufferers will most likely suffer from it again in a year, and with time, the attacks might even last longer, involve more of the joints, and become a lot more frequent.

An example of an instance of gout is that you may fall asleep at night in a perfectly healthy condition, only to wake you in the middle of the night with a sharp pain, most probably in your big toe. Sometimes, this pain could even be felt in the ankle, instep, or heel. The sensation or the pain that you will feel due to gout will be so acute that the bed sheet weight on the toe will also not be tolerable for you. The intensity and the persistence of the pain are extremely high.

The joint that is known to be affected in most cases is that of the base of the big toe. However, this does not necessarily mean that no other joint can be affected. Your lower limb joints can also be involved in this case. Due to gout, the tendons and the bursa can also be affected. This causes swelling of the soft tissue

5

underneath the joint of the elbow, for example. The soft tissues that surround the affected joint can become hot, swollen, and red. Eventually, this swelling can affect the entire ankle, or foot which will be a huge hindrance since you will not even be able to wear your shoes on the toe, ankle, or foot that is inflamed.

Chronic Gout

Chronic gout is the most excessive form of gout, and this stage arises after years and only after a person does not receive the proper medical attention that they need in order to recover. In some cases, gout attacks that have been left untreated can linger and this disease can become chronic, which results in inflammation on a persistent basis. In this case, the uric acid crystals will deposit in as well as around the joint. This can lead to a destruction of the soft tissues surrounding the joint and the joint itself. When such a thing happens, this is known as tophaceous gout. However, if people were to receive proper treatment for gout, they would never progress through such an advanced stage of gout.

5. What Is Uric Acid?

Uric acid is a waste product that needs to be eliminated by the body through urination. It is developed from the breakdown of a substance called purines that are known to be present in many of the foods that we consume in our everyday lives. When uric acid is formed, it normally dissolves within the blood and passes through the kidneys and into the urine. This is how it gets eliminated. However, if this uric acid is produced in excessive amounts or if the kidneys do not remove sufficient uric acid from the system, this can result in a significant build-up within the blood. This condition is known as hyperuricemia. The condition can arise when foods rich in purines have been consumed. While hyperuricemia is not dangerous, excessive crystals of uric acid can be formed as a result of this, thus leading to gout. These crystals can then deposit within the joints and cause inflammation.

The next page shows a flowchart explaining how gout develops in an easy and compressed manner.

6. A Flowchart Explaining How Gout Develops

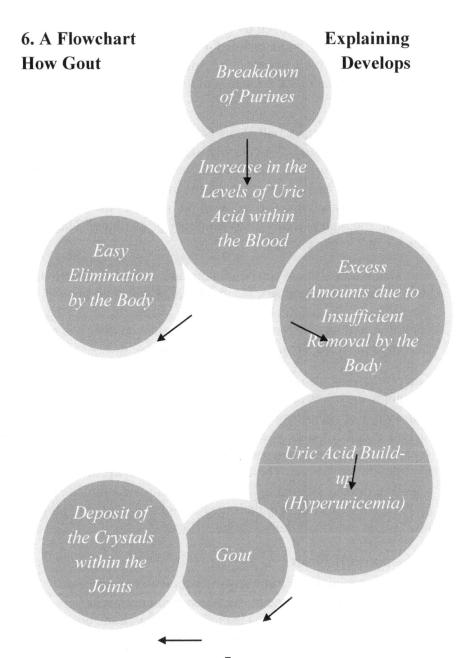

Breakdown of Purines

Increase in the Levels of Uric Acid within the Blood

Easy Elimination by the Body

Excess Amounts due to Insufficient Removal by the Body

Uric Acid Build-up (Hyperuricemia)

Deposit of the Crystals within the Joints

Gout

Chapter 2: Gout In Detail

1. Characteristics Of Gout

The disease is characterized by severe, sharp, and sudden tenderness, redness, and attacks of pain in the joints, particularly the joint located at the big toe. The pain is caused by the needle-like crystal formation of the uric acid that is deposited in the joints.

An acute pain or attack will also wake you up from sleep because of the burning sensation in your big toe. Since the affected joint is so tender and swollen, even placing a sheet on it will be intolerable. For many of the people, the initial symptom of gout is a lot of pain accompanied by swelling in the big toe, and this swelling and pain is followed by an injury or an illness. The attack can become chronic.

Fortunately, the disease can be treated, and it should be treated as soon as the sensation arises. If left untreated, the condition can permanently damage the kidneys and the joints. However, the condition will only become this severe if a person does not seek treatment for it for a consecutive 10 years or so.

The crystals can also eventually develop in the skin that surrounds the joints or cause stones in kidneys. There are also many ways of significantly reducing the occurrence of the disease. There are also other health risks associated with gout such as diabetes, cardiovascular disease, high blood pressure, and chronic kidney disease. Therefore, someone with the disease or who is at the risk of getting it should maintain a healthy lifestyle by exercising, maintaining their ideal weight, and incorporating a healthy diet into their daily routine.

2. Causes Of Gout

As we have seen, the initial cause of gout is the presence of excess uric acid within the blood, a condition known as hyperuricemia. This uric acid is produced through the breakdown of purines within the body. Purines are compounds found in specific food items such as seafood, poultry, meat, mushrooms, dried beans, liver, mackerel, and anchovies. However, when the waste product uric acid is formed it needs to be eliminated by the kidneys and through the urine. In some cases, more uric acid is produced than is eliminated, leading to a build-up inside the body. This build-up then forms needle-like crystals, leading to pain and inflammation of the joint and the surrounding tissue. There are a few factors that increase the chances of a person being affected by gout. These factors are listed below:

Gender And Age

Men have a higher chance of being affected by the disease since they tend to produce more uric acid compared to women. However, the chances of women being affected by gout increases after menopause, as then the uric acid levels in women increase and become the same as that of men.

Genetics

If you have a history of gout within your family, then you might have an increased likelihood of contracting the disease, and therefore, should take more precaution.

Lifestyle

If you are at a higher risk of developing gout you should limit your consumption of alcohol and purine intake. The more alcohol you consume, the harder your body will have to work to remove uric acid from your body. Also, since purines are broken down into uric acid, the higher the purines you consume in your diet, the more the chances of the uric acid concentration increasing in your body.

Exposure To lead

Chronic exposure to lead is not good and has been linked in some cases to the occurrence of gout. Lead is also known to cause many other health problems. Therefore, it is best to stay away from it.

Medications

Certain types of medications can cause an increase in the levels of uric acid within the body. These medications include drugs and diuretics that contain salicylate.

Weight

If you are overweight you can significantly increase your chances of getting gout, as the body contains more tissue that can be broken down, thus resulting in the excessive production of uric acid. This is not all. Being overweight leads to a lot of other medical-related issues as well.

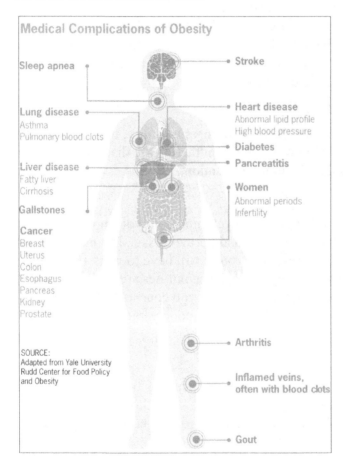

Medical Complications of Obesity

Sleep apnea

Stroke

Lung disease
Asthma
Pulmonary blood clots

Heart disease
Abnormal lipid profile
High blood pressure

Diabetes

Liver disease
Fatty liver
Cirrhosis

Pancreatitis

Gallstones

Women
Abnormal periods
Infertility

Cancer
Breast
Uterus
Colon
Esophagus
Pancreas
Kidney
Prostate

SOURCE:
Adapted from Yale University
Rudd Center for Food Policy
and Obesity

Arthritis

Inflamed veins,
often with blood clots

Gout

Source: www.Wikipedia.org

Other Issues Related To Health

If the kidneys remain inefficient at the removal of adequate amounts of waste products, the levels of uric acid can increase. Other conditions such as diabetes, hypothyroidism, and high blood pressure can also result in gout.

3. Signs And Symptoms

Symptoms of gout can arise unexpectedly and without much warning. The main signs and symptoms of gout include:

Intense Amount Of Joint Pain

In most cases, gout will affect the large joint of the big toe. However, gout symptoms could also appear in the ankles, wrists, hands, and feet. The most severe pain that I experienced is during the first 12 to 24 hours right after gout begins.

Lingering Discomfort

There might be some lingering joint discomfort or pain after the most severe pain has passed. This lingering pain could last for a few days or even a few weeks. The attacks that happen later could last even longer and affect even more joints.

Redness And Inflammation

Another sign of gout is that the joints that are affected become tender, red, and swollen.

4. Stages Of Gout Progression

A grout typically progresses through four stages. Each of these stages has its own signs and symptoms that it is characterized by.

Asymptomatic Hyperuricemia

A person can be affected by hyperuricemia without even having any outward symptoms. This is an early stage of gout where treatment might not be necessary. However, the urate crystals still get deposited within tissues and this can cause a little damage within the body.

Acute Gout

This is the stage where the urate crystals that were being deposited in the earlier stage of asymptomatic hyperuricemia cause intense pain and acute inflammation all of a sudden. This sudden attack is called a flare, and will normally die down within the next three to ten days. Alcohol, drugs, or stressful conditions and events can also trigger flares.

Interval Or Inter Critical Gout

This stage happens between the acute gout attacks. The flares that could arise after the initial ones might not occur for the next few months or even years. However, if these flares are not treated, they can last even longer and occur on a more frequent basis. This is also the stage where more of the urate crystals will get deposited within the tissues.

Chronic Tophaceous Gout

The final stage of gout is perhaps the worst of all the stages. This is where permanent damage can be caused to the kidneys and joints. The patient can also develop tophi (huge lumps of rate crystals) in the regions of the body that are much cooler than the rest such as the finger joints, or even get chronic arthritis.

The chronic tophaceous gout stage is only reached if a patient does not get their gout treated for a long time, such as 10 years or so. A patient will unlikely ever reach this stage if they receive proper treatment and on time.

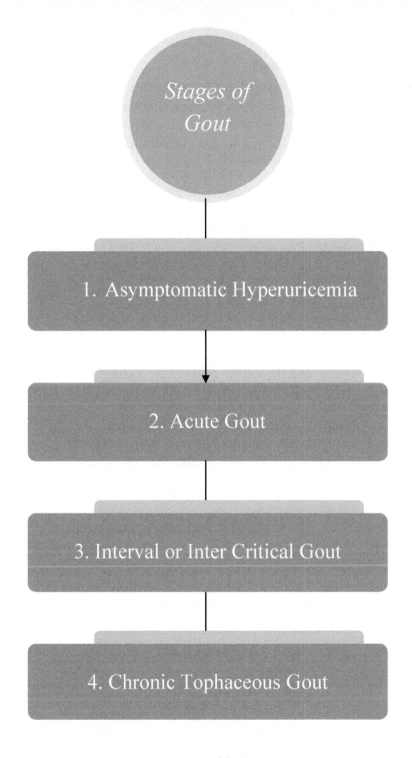

Stages of Gout

1. Asymptomatic Hyperuricemia

2. Acute Gout

3. Interval or Inter Critical Gout

4. Chronic Tophaceous Gout

5. Tests And Diagnosis

While gout results in very distinctive and painful symptoms, especially during flare-ups, the condition is not always easy to diagnose. In addition, in some instances the symptoms can be pretty vague. Gout symptoms are also sometimes similar to the symptoms of other conditions.

Take the example of hyperuricemia. While this condition can occur in most people that develop the disease, it might not occur during a flare. Most of the people who develop hyperuricemia might not even develop gout.

There are normally two diagnostic tests performed by doctors in order to find out whether a person has gout or not. These are as follows:

Joint Fluid Test

The joint fluid test consists of the extraction of fluid with the help of a needle from the joint that has been affected. This fluid will then be examined to check whether or not there are any urate crystals present within the fluid. Some joint infections can also cause symptoms that are similar to gout. However, in these conditions, a doctor can look for the presence of bacteria so that the condition can be ruled out.

Blood Test

A blood test can also be carried out in order to measure the uric acid levels within the blood. However, one thing to keep in mind is that not everyone with high levels of uric acid will experience the condition. On the other hand, some people can develop the condition without the increased amounts of uric acid within their blood.

A condition that is often confused with that of gout is called pseudogout. This condition presents symptoms that are very similar to those of gout. However, a major difference is that in pseudogout the joints are irritated by the calcium phosphate crystals as opposed to the urate crystals. Since the crystals are different, both conditions would require different modes of treatment.

6. Ways To Lower The Risk Of Gout

Maintain A Healthy Weight
Being overweight does not help when you have the risk of getting gout. Therefore, you need to lose the excess amount of weight. This is because the excessive amounts of body tissue would result in the production of extra amounts of uric acid. You can seek help from your doctor with regards to a proper weight plan and goal. Get started with regular exercise. Low impact and gentle forms of exercise are best for those suffering from arthritis. You should also consume food that have controlled amounts of calories, especially plant foods like vegetables. Increase your consumption of low fat dairy products and consume moderate amounts of lean protein.

Avoid Meats Rich In Purine And Seafood
Purine is known to increase the amount of uric acid within the body, and if you suffer from gout, then diets rich in purine can be bad for you. Seafood can also increase the levels of uric acid within the body. However, vegetables rich in purine are perfectly fine to consume since they do not increase the levels of uric acid within the body.

Choose Dairy Products Low In Fat
If you consume yogurt and milk that consist of a reduced fat content, then you can ensure a significant reduction in your risk of getting gout. Therefore, be sure to add some fat free or reduced fat yogurt and milk to your diet. These two items are also rich in vitamin D, thereby helping to improve the health of your joints and increase your muscular strength significantly.

Reduce Your Intake Of Alcohol (Especially Beer)
Alcoholic beverages are bad for people who are at an increased risk of getting gout, since these beverages hinder the ability of the body to clear out the uric acid. Beer is probably the worst of all

the alcoholic beverages, as according to Harvard researchers, men who consumed two or more beers on a daily basis were twice as likely to suffer from the condition compared to men who did not have any beer at all. Spirits also result in increased chances of getting gout, however this is still less than the threat that beer presents. Wine does not increase the gout risk. However, it is still better to reduce the consumption of wine.

Avoid The Consumption Of Sugary Beverages
Fructose is a type of sugar that has the potential of increasing the risk of gout by increasing the levels of uric acid within the blood. This type of sugar is found in all of the soft drinks and sweetened beverages, as well as other food such as cookies, candy, and baked goods. A study conducted in 2008 found that men who consumed high amounts of fructose had twice as much chance of developing gout as opposed to men who did not consume that much fructose. It is best to reduce your sugar and sweetener intake, especially those sugars containing about 90% fructose.

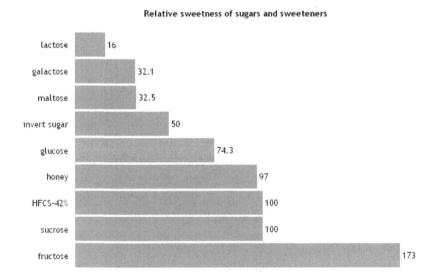

Relative sweetness of sugars and sweeteners

lactose	16
galactose	32.1
maltose	32.5
invert sugar	50
glucose	74.3
honey	97
HFCS-42%	100
sucrose	100
fructose	173

Source: www.Wikipedia.org

Drink Lots of Water

People who suffer from gout should significantly increase their water intake and drink at least 8 glasses daily. This will help to flush out excess uric acid from the body along with all the other toxins that accumulate on a daily basis. Water not only keeps you hydrated, it is also the best choice of beverage since it contains no sugar, calories, or artificial sweeteners and ingredients. It is very refreshing and completely natural.

Use Aspirin Only Sparingly

Aspirin contains active ingredients by the name of salicylates. These active ingredients can significantly increase the levels of uric acid within the blood. Therefore, consuming aspirin or related products is a bad idea for those people who already have gout or are at a risk of developing gout. In addition, in case you require painkillers, you should talk to your doctor and find out about other pain relievers that you can safely take.

Get a Check-up

Apart from all of the points mentioned above, you should make it a point to visit your doctor on a regular basis so that you can get your overall health checked. This will also allow your doctor to run tests for gout in case you are at an increased risk of contracting that disease.

You should also know that about 75% of the people who are diagnosed with gout also develop a metabolic syndrome. This metabolic syndrome increases the risk of getting heart disease, and it is therefore a very serious condition. Hence if your doctor gives you a diagnosis of gout, then ask him to run tests for metabolic syndrome as well.

Chapter 3: Diet And Recipes For Gout

1. The Best Traditional Cure For Gout: Diet

Treatments

One of the best possible treatments for gout involves the use of specific food items that have low levels of purines and help in reducing the overall levels of uric acid within the body.

Some of the food items that have shown amazingly positive results in reducing the levels of uric acid or the overall symptoms related to gout are celery, bing cherries, a lot of water, and cheese. Dehydration is a huge negative factor when it comes to the proper functioning of the kidneys and as a result can cause a build-up of uric acid within the body. When you consume water, which is slightly towards the alkaline side, it can help in reducing the acidity in the body.

An individual must also avoid carbonated and sugary drinks since they also considerably increase the risk of gout. Instead of drinking carbonated beverages, a person should consume fruit juices. The usual suspects for gout must obviously be avoided. These include foods rich in protein, seafood such as sardines, cauliflower, asparagus, spinach, mushrooms, meats, dry beans, and especially alcohol. Some of these foods however, particularly those coming from a plant, can be eaten on an occasional basis, since the purines found in plants are not as harmful as those found in animal-related products. However, be sure to talk to your doctor and make a proper diet plan for yourself so that you do not end up overdoing it on one particular item.

Purines also get broken down into uric acid. Therefore, people who are at a significant risk of developing gout, or who already have it, should avoid a diet that is rich in purines. Once you change your diet according to your personal needs and requirements, you will feel that any incidences of future gout attacks will be considerably reduced and you will be able to lead a much happier life.

There is still a lot of inconsistency when it comes to food recommended by various doctors and nutritionists for gout patients. Some might recommend one thing while others might recommend something totally different. However, there is one thing that all of them will agree upon, and that is the importance of maintaining and having an ideal body weight. In case you are overweight, you should take steps to reduce that extra weight and fat instantly. This can be done with the help of a health program and making sure that you are getting enough exercise on a regular basis. However, be sure that you do everything in a slow and gradual manner since a crash diet can significantly increase the uric acid levels within your blood. You should be extra careful when it comes to gout, and be sure that you do not end up taking extreme steps.

A healthy diet is a great way to make you feel more effective by giving you a lot more energy and keeping your stress levels down. Be sure to note what you are eating though. If you consume too many purines, then it can lead to a negative consequence for you. Fat content in the foods that you consume should also be low, and especially keep a watchful eye on cholesterol and saturated fat.

Alcohol is a big NO when it comes to treating and taking care of gout. Consuming alcohol, particularly beer, can cause dehydration and prevent the uric acid in the body from being eliminated effectively. This can eventually lead to gout, especially if you are highly prone to it. You should instead consume a lot of fluids to help make the uric acid present within the urine and blood more dilute. Vitamin C can also be hugely beneficial in the management and prevention of gout and other diseases associated with urates.

2. Delicious Recipes That Are Great For Gout

In case you have gout, staying away from too much alcohol, bread, or food rich in purines is the best thing to do. These food items include red meat and seafood. While it may seem that people who have gout do not have much to eat, it is not all that bad once you get a little creative with the ingredients that you can consume. Here are a few recipes that you should definitely try if you have gout:

Sweet Potato, Ginger And Carrot Soup

This soup will make a great comfort food for you during the winters, especially if you have gout. Sweet potatoes, spices and carrots do not contain huge amounts of purines, thereby making this soup ideal for gout patients. You can make this soup even more in line with your condition if you use a vegetable stock instead of using chicken broth.

Updated Waldorf Salad

For this salad, you can make use of mayonnaise that is low in fat along with dried cranberries, grapes, walnuts, celery, and apples. The crunchy salad will help to replenish your hunger in the best of ways. Not only are the ingredients low in purines, the cranberries, apples, and grapes also contain a rich amount of malic acid that may help in reducing the levels of uric acid within the body.

Goat's Cheese and Eggplant Sandwich

Tomatoes and eggplant in this sandwich are both extremely low in purines. Along with this, the ingredients blend in a highly delicious manner with the goat's cheese, which has a very creamy texture. Such a combination of ingredients will definitely not be something boring to eat.

The inclusion of vegetables in this sandwich is most likely to help in neutralizing the uric acid within the body, since vegetables are more alkaline in nature.

Tomato Crostini

This recipe is perfect even if you have guests coming over. The appetizer consists of plum tomatoes that are far better than some of the other varieties during the winter season.

Lemon And Sage Roasted Chicken

While it is true that people who have gout should not consume meat, it is also true that this food cannot be avoided in all instances. However, people who suffer from gout can opt for chicken or duck instead of turkey, pork, or red meat since these consist of fewer amounts of purines.

The recipe is extremely easy to make and the flavours of the chicken are enhanced further with the sage and lemon that is used. The carrots, turnips, and parsnips that are used on the side are great in flavour and very low in purines.

Blood Orange And Duck Confit Salad

This highly special salad is low in purines. Thus, it will never aggravate your gout-related conditions, yet it will satisfy your hunger for meat. Duck is a better option when it comes to meat, while oranges contain a lot of vitamin C and according to research vitamin C is great when it comes to lowering the levels of uric acid within the body. The other ingredients in this dish include hazelnuts, vinegar, and oil, which are all low in purines.

Zucchini Spaghetti

Pasta is a great food that is low in purines and fills you up instantly without putting meat in it. The roasted jalapenos and zucchini in the dish help to give it an additional touch of amazing taste.

However, be sure that you do not end up eating a lot of it. After all, you would not want to become overweight, especially if you have or are at a high risk of developing gout. The calories in this food are already a considerable amount and therefore your serving size should be small.

Rosemary Roasted Potatoes

Potatoes are another great option for a dish that is low in purines and high in vitamin C, in addition to the fact that the uric acid levels within the body are reduced. Fresh rosemary further helps to add to the overall flavour of the dish and is also considered to be great for blood circulation. This benefit can really help in the easing of the inflammation and pain associated with gout.

Vanilla Bean Pudding

While many of the recipes required to make milk and chocolate pudding use whole and thick milk, this recipe can substitute the traditional milk with some skimmed milk that is fat free. This substitution will be a lot better for people who suffer from gout. Plus, the great aspect about the dish is that despite minimising the amount of fat used, the flavour of the dish will remain the same.

Peaches And Berry Sauce

Instead of using the traditional chocolate syrup, you can make use of some berry sauce for a delicious vanilla ice cream that is low in fat. Dark berries are known to be great for lowing the levels of uric acid within the body, just like blackberries.

Apart from this, fruits such as berries and peaches are also used in this dessert item that are both low in purines and delicious at the same time.

Raspberry Tarts

This little dessert is rich in delicious flavour and low in dairy fat. The raspberry used in this dessert is also great for patients looking after their gout.

Pumpkin Pancakes

A pumpkin pie will be full of calories and this can make you fat if you end up eating too much of it. Being overweight is not good, especially if you have or are at risk of developing gout. However, you can try some pumpkin pancakes that use not that many pumpkins, and hence you will end up consuming fewer calories.

Cornflakes In Low Fat Milk With Berries

You can start your mornings with some delicious and healthy cereal mixed with nutritious berries. This meal will be rich in fibre and antioxidants and is also perfect for people who suffer from gout.

Some research that was conducted suggested that dairy that is low in fat could help decrease the gout risk significantly. Dairy products are also known to be rich in protein and they could be a great alternative for meat, especially for people who have gout.

These are just some of the great and delicious recipes for people who have gout. While these people may think that they do not have many options when it comes to eating food, they are not aware that with the right kind of mixing and matching, they can come up with some of the most delicious alternatives. When they eat right and take care of the amount of calories they consume, they will automatically start feeling healthier and happier.

Chapter 4: Treatment And Prevention

1. General Measures For Self Help

If you suffer from gout you are most likely to develop swelling and redness in the region where your joints have been affected. You can, however, take certain measures to reduce this swelling by raising the limb that has been affected, provided that you are able to do this. This limb will most probably be your leg. If you cannot raise your leg on your own, then you can ask someone around you to help you out. A very easy way to raise your limb is to lie on a sofa and place your leg on a cushion. Place an ice pack or a frozen pack or peas against the joint that is inflamed so that you can ease your pain significantly, at least until the pain and treatment medications for gout start doing their job.

In case you are making use of an ice pack, be sure to wrap it in a towel so that direct contact of this ice pack with the skin can be avoided. Direct contact can result in an ice burn and you would not want that. Only apply this ice pack for 20 minutes or so since you should avoid using it for a long period of time. After the first 20 minutes are up and you have given some time for the temperature of that region of your limb to return back to normal, you may reapply the ice pack.

You should also consider using a cane or some type of support if you have to walk around. This is especially true in cases where your joint is swollen and red. A cane or a support will assist you in keeping an unnecessary amount of weight off your affected joint. You should also be sure to drink lots of water to stay hydrated so that the intensity and frequency of your future attacks can be minimized. Cherry juice and taking vitamin C supplements also help greatly in decreasing the severity and intensity of future attacks.

2. Medications And Other Treatments

The treatment of gout normally involves the use of various types of medications. Your doctor, on the basis of your preferences and current health, will give these medications to you. These medications are used to treat a variety of conditions. These conditions include:

- Future flares
- Complications from gout such as developing tophi and kidney stones
- Gout attacks

Some of the commonly used medications are described in detail in the next section. These medications help to reduce the pain and inflammation in the areas of the body that have been affected and are usually administered orally.

The medications either help to improve the ability of the kidney to remove the excess amounts of uric acid from the body or to reduce the uric acid production in general. There are also many dietary and lifestyle choices and guidelines that a person can follow in order to protect themselves against the occurrence of gout or future flares. These guidelines have been mentioned in the previous chapters. If you are looking to lose weight, then avoid diets that contain low amounts of carbohydrate. This is because when the level of carbohydrate in the body is insufficient, the body will not be able to burn its fat properly. This, in turn, will release ketones into the blood stream, a substance that is known to increase the uric acid levels within the blood.

3. Medications That Help In Treating Gout Attacks

The medications that are used to prevent future gout attacks or treat acute attacks include:

Allopurinol

Allopurinol is most commonly used in the treatment and control of gout by making sure that the purine levels are kept to a minimum. This means that the medication needs to be taken for the long run. Unfortunately, there are sometimes serious side effects of the drug. These side effects include Stevens-Johnson syndrome, which is a painful and life-threatening condition that involves mucus membranes, as well as other hypersensitivity reactions that are similar in nature.

Allopurinol should not be used to lower uric acid levels. The drug should only be taken in instances where you have to keep gout under control once it occurs. You should also keep in mind that when you first start taking allopurinol, the gout attacks may increase and not lessen during the first few months. Many doctors might not even recommend this medication, so be sure to consult your doctor before having it.

Allopurinol is sometimes also prescribed to patients who have kidney stones or cancer. It is an inhibitor that prevents the xanthine oxidase release. This compound helps in the formation of uric acid.

The drug has been used within the US since 1964. Initially, it was used in the treatment of infections, ulcers, and seizures, for the improvement of survival chances when a person has had bypass surgery, and for the prevention of kidney rejection in cases where patients have had a kidney transplant.

Some of the side effects of allopurinol include drowsiness, indigestion, vomiting, nausea, diarrhoea, upset stomach, eye irritation, mouth and lip swelling, chills, sore throat, fever, skin rashes, bloody urine or stool, and painful urination. Other more serious side effects of the drug include bone marrow failure in producing blood cells, blood vessel inflammation, and liver inflammation. It is also important to note that allopurinol has the tendency of interfering with other medications, thereby reducing effectiveness and increasing toxicity.

Nonsteroidal Anti-Inflammatory Drugs (NSAIDs)
NSAIDs help in controlling pain and inflammation in people who suffer from gout. Your doctor may prescribe a higher dose in order to stop acute attacks. This could be followed by a lower dose on a daily basis to prevent and save a person from future attacks. NSAIDs typically include certain over the counter

medications such as naproxen (Aleve) and ibuprofen (Motrin, Advil), as well as prescriptions that are more powerful like indomethacin (indocin). These medications do however carry a risk of ulcers, stomach pain, and bleeding.

Colchicine

If you cannot take NSAIDs for some reason, then your doctor can advise you to take colchicine (Colcrys). This is a kind of pain reliever that helps to reduce gout pain very effectively, especially when the medication is taken as soon as the pain or the symptoms start. This drug also has some side effects, which can be intolerable. These side effects include vomiting, diarrhoea, and nausea. After the resolution of the acute attacks from the disease, your doctor may ask you to take lower doses of the medication on a daily basis so that future attacks can be prevented.

Corticosteroids

These medications, like the drug named prednisone, help in controlling the pain and inflammation that result because of gout. These pills may be taken orally or injected into the joint. Your doctor can inject this medication into your joint when you come in for the joint fluid test. Corticosteroids are normally only taken by people who cannot consume colchicines or NSAIDs.

Some of the side effects of this drug may include decreased infection fighting abilities, poor healing of wounds, and thinning of the bones. In order to reduce the risk of getting these side effects, your doctor will try to prescribe you the lowest dose that keeps your symptoms under control, and also prescribe you with steroids for as short a time as possible.

Probenicid

Probenicid helps in the excretion of more uric acid. However, you should only take this medication if your kidneys are healthy, functioning well, and are able to excrete the excessive uric acid. Unfortunately, the medication might also cause kidney stones and you should refrain from taking this if you are using aspirin or diuretics.

27

Sulfinpyrazone

This also helps in reducing the uric acid quantity within the blood. However, it can make you feel sick in the process. The side effects of this type of drug include vomiting, nausea, and diarrhoea. It might also cause a significant increase in the effect of blood thinners. It is due to this reason you should not be taking sulfinpyrazone with NSAIDs or aspirin.

It is important that you consult your doctor before taking any of the above-mentioned gout medication, especially since some of them have very serious side effects.

4. Prevention

While some of the risk factors that are associated with gout may be genetic, there are still others that are not genetic. The genetic risks might not be preventable. However, you can always make some changes in your lifestyle to reduce its occurrence significantly such as taking care of your diet and taking care of obesity. Many people can prevent the occurrence of gout by simply following a healthy diet and maintaining a healthy weight. Once again, your diet should consist of low amounts of refined carbohydrates along with red meat and saturated fats.

Sufficient fluid intake is also very important when it comes to the prevention of gout and attacks. This also helps to decrease the risk of the formation of kidney stones, especially in people who suffer from gout. Consuming less alcohol will also be beneficial, since alcohol is a diuretic that can contribute to dehydration, leading to acute attacks of gout. Alcohol also results in hyperuricemia, since it affects the metabolism of uric acid. It results in uric acid being excreted by the body at a very slow pace. This forms uric acid crystals within the joints and also causes dehydration.

Certain dietary changes can also help you to prevent gout completely, especially if you are at a higher risk of getting it, or reduce the amount of uric acid within the blood. You can start off by avoiding foods that are rich in purines. In addition, if you happen to be overweight, then take steps to reduce the excess fat on your body and keep yourself fit.

5. Medications That Help To Prevent Complications From Gout

If you happen to experience gout attacks on a less frequent basis but which happen to be more painful, or if you get many gout attacks in a year, then your doctor might prescribe you certain medications in order to reduce your risk of getting complications related to the disease. Some of the options of these medications include:

Medications That Aid In The Blockage Of Uric Acid Production
The drugs that are known as xanthine oxidase inhibitors and that include febuxostat (Uloric) and allopurinol (Aloprim, Zyloprim, Lopurin) are known to limit the uric acid amounts that your body ends up making. This will significantly help in lowering the levels of uric acid in your blood and hence reduce the risk of getting gout. Some of the side effects of allopurinol include low blood count and rashes. The side effects of febuxostat on the other hand include nausea, reduced functioning of the liver, and rashes.

Xanthine oxidase inhibitors can also trigger a completely new and acute attack if these are taken before the complete resolution of any recent attacks. However, if you happen to take a short course of colchicines on a low dose before you start off with xanthine oxidase inhibitor, then this can significantly reduce such risks.

Medication That Improves The Removal Of Uric Acid
Probenecid (Probalan) is one such type of medication that improves that ability of the kidneys in the removal of uric acid from your body. This helps to significantly lower the levels of uric acid within your body and hence reduce your risk of getting gout. However, this medication increases the levels of uric acid that are passed through your urine. Some of the side effects that

people can get from this medication include kidney stones, stomach pain, and rashes.

6. Alternative Medicine For Treating Gout

If you feel that your gout treatments are not working as well as you had hoped, you might want to look at some alternative treatment options. However, before you get into this, you should speak to your doctor so that you can weigh up the risks and benefits of each of these options before you choose the right treatment for yourself. There are certain food items or nutrients that have been known to reduce the levels of uric acid within the system. These include:

Coffee

There have been some studies conducted that show a link between regularly drinking coffee (both decaffeinated and regular coffee) and lower levels of uric acid. However, there has been no study that shows why or how coffee has this kind of an effect.

Vitamin C

Supplements that contain Vitamin C are known to reduce the uric acid levels within the body. However, this nutrient has not been studied well enough to be sure of how it helps in treating gout. Be careful of taking in too much vitamin C since that has the potential of increasing the levels of uric acid within the body. Be sure to speak to your doctor so that they can provide you with a reasonable dosage of vitamin C. Always remember that the best way to consume vitamin C is through fruits and vegetables, especially oranges.

Cherries

In many studies, cherries have been known to lower the uric acid levels within the body. However, there is no clear evidence whether they have any effect on the signs and symptoms of gout. Eating cherries and some other fruits such as blueberries, raspberries, purple grapes, and blackberries, may be a great way of treating gout. However, have a discussion with your doctor regarding this.

There are many other alternative or complementary medicine treatments that help you with your gout pain. For example, certain relaxation techniques such as meditation and deep breathing exercises can provide aid in taking your mind off the condition and the pain.

7. Natural Medicines And Their Effect On Gout

Many people would wonder whether natural medicines would have any effect on their gout. However, with the amount of pain that they experience, these people end up taking these natural medicines anyway.

You might even see a lot of adverts all around you by the people who sell natural cures stating that these cures are far better at treating gout than the treatments that the doctors prescribe to patients. The idea of treating gout with the help of natural medications seems like a really good idea for all those people who have not been finding any kind of relief from their medication.

Natural medicines are made from herbal extracts and have no association with the FDA (Food and Drug Administration). All these medicines also claim that they have no side effects whatsoever and happen to be quite expensive. Here are a few of the natural medications that are available in the market:

Milk Thistle (silymarin)
This helps in liver production and the growth of new liver cells. The herb has a negative effect if taken with phenytoin, halothane, and antipsychotics, and might have enhancing effects of aspirin in case of liver damage. This could lead to an overdose of aspirin. A person might consider using it for certain chemotherapies and in the conditions of cirrhosis, inflammation of the liver, or hepatitis.

Milk thistle grows all around the world and is found in dry and sunny places in most cases. It has a long stem of about 4 to 10 feet and has wide leaves.

A special chemical in milk thistle known as silymarin assists in the protection of liver cells. It achieves this in three unique ways:

- Silymarin consists of anti-inflammatory properties that help in ensuring that the cells of the liver do not swell up when injured.
- The growth of liver cells is also encouraged. This helps in stopping the toxins from reaching the liver cells.
- The antioxidant properties of the chemical help in protecting the cells from getting damaged. This damage will normally be caused due to oxidation.

Recent research also suggests that milk thistle helps to keep the liver well protected. In fact, it actually helps in relieving the symptoms of certain inflammatory conditions such as gout, cirrhosis, and hepatitis.

Milk thistle will also heal and protect the liver from any damage caused by diseases, alcohol, toxic plants, chemicals and drugs.

Scientists are now also looking at the effect of milk thistle on skin cancer, allergies, and high cholesterol. Milk thistle is also found to be injected in people who have consumed poisonous mushrooms. This will act as an antidote. Scientists are now also looking for ways that this product will help in decreasing the damage to the liver that is caused as a result of chemotherapy. Many people think that the herb is great at helping the body rid all the toxins much more effectively.

Milk thistle is found in the form of tablets, capsules, soft gels, and tinctures. In case you want to use the herb for treating problems with the liver, around 400 to 600 mg of the herb should be taken throughout the day in equal doses.

However, if you want to use milk thistle be sure to ask your doctor. This will make sure that the herb will not interfere with other medications that you might be consuming.

While milk thistle does not have any side effects, it should only be consumed according to the recommended dosage. You must also know that while the toxins are being released from the body you might have to go through feelings of pain, bloating, diarrhoea, headache, skin reactions, rare cases of anaphylaxis, rhino conjunctivitis and changes in bowel movements.

Milk thistle is easily available from the grocery and health food stores that are selling herbal and vitamin supplements. However, be sure that you read the label so that you can be sure that you are only consuming legitimate milk thistle supplement and nothing else. After all, you do not want to end up consuming harmful chemicals and products.

Aged Garlic (sativum)

This is great for detoxification. It does not even have any side effects unless you want to take into account the bad breath that it causes. Aged garlic is great for your health and can easily be added to one's diet.

Yucca Stalk (saponins)

This is great for the mobilization of purines. Yucca has been a very popular treatment for gout amongst Native Americans. However, the ingredient can also cause diarrhoea. If it is constantly used over longer periods of time, it can prevent the adequate absorption of fat-soluble vitamins such as vitamins A, D, E, and K. There are no drug interactions that are known for Yucca Stalk.

Artichoke Powder

Artichoke powder is used for the production of bile and there are no side effects of this substance as far as researchers know. You can consider adding artichokes to a salad that you prepare for yourself to get the same amount of benefits that you will receive from the artichoke powder.

Turmeric

Turmeric is great as it offers protection to the liver and has amazing anti-inflammatory properties. The ingredient is also used a lot in Asia and India to flavour food. It is great at helping cancer patients when they are undergoing chemotherapy. Some of the medical literature though suggests that Turmeric can cause the development of gallstones.

Before taking these natural medicines though, you should have a word with your doctor regarding the feasibility of that medicine. This recommendation from your doctor will help you to make a much better and informed decision so that you do not have to suffer from any unexpected or nasty side effects.

8. Two Herbs That Can Do Wonders For People With Gout

a) Celery Seed

Celery seed is not only meant for soups and salads, but can also be used as a medicinal herb. The seeds of celery appear on the plant after the flowers start being produced. In many parts of the world, celery seed has been considered to be a medicinal remedy for a long time. The harvesting of the seeds begins in the second years of the plant. The stalks and seeds of celery are known to consist of many essential compounds such as vitamins A, C, E, and K, along with many important minerals i.e. iron, magnesium, manganese, phosphorus, calcium, amino acids, essential oils, as well as a sedative known as phthalide. Apart from the treatment of gout, celery seed is also known to be amazing for indigestion and arthritis.

History Of Celery Seed

Ancient Egyptians made use of celery as food. The leaves of celery were made into garlands and placed in King Tutankhamen's tomb. Ancient Greeks and Romans also made use of celery for medicinal and food purposes. Some people from the ancient era even considered Celery to be an aphrodisiac.

Aulus Cornelius Celcus from Rome found in 30 AD that celery seeds could be used in the treatment of inflammation and pain. Celery seeds were also made use of for the rituals and ceremonies that dealt with the underworld and death.

The Herbalist Nicholas Culpeper, who was situated in Europe, mentioned in 1653 that celery seeds had the power of purifying and sweetening the human blood.

Ailments That Are Cured By Celery Seeds

- Anti-inflammatory qualities help with the conditions of gout, rheumatoid arthritis, neuralgia, and osteoarthritis
- Increases and breaks down the excretions of uric acid, which relieves gout pain
- Helps to calm the digestive system
- Eases joint pain that often results from degeneration as a result of aging and inflammation
- Essential oils can help to reduce muscle spasms and inflammation
- Increases the appetite
- May relieve pain due to arthritis
- Oil may also help to calm the nerves
- Promotes the individual's cardiac health
- Promotes the urine flow due to the diuretic properties that help in the flushing out of excess fluids and toxins
- Relieves bladder problems like urinary tract infections and cystitis
- Relieves gas and indigestion
- Relieves kidney disorders like gravel and stones

Celery Seeds And The Treatment Of Gout

Celery seeds can act as a great diuretic. Due to this reason, it is often used for the treatment of gout. The seeds are not only helpful in the case of the retention of fluids, but also help in the flushing out of the needle-like crystals of uric acid. These are the main causes of why gout arises in the first place. Celery seeds also consist of antiseptic compounds that are great at easing urinary tract inflammation, as a result of which significant discomfort can arise. The herb is also great at ensuring a healthy overall bodily system. Celery seed extract can also be used instead of Allopurinol, which is a pharmaceutical drug that also helps in getting rid of uric acid from the body. If a person consumes 2 to 4 celery seed extract tablets each day, then they can benefit from the prevention of future gout attacks. The use of celery seed extract will even help in avoiding the adverse side effects that the drug Allopurinol can have on a person, since you will no longer feel the need to take it.

Other Celery Seed Uses

The oil that is extracted from celery seed is used by the pharmaceutical and perfume industries. It is also used for seasoning in culinary dishes or even mixed with some sea salt to transform it into celery salt.

Precautions

Women who are pregnant should stay away from the remedies involving celery seeds. The general use of celery seeds should also be such that the dosage needs to be low. This is because the seeds can cause photosensitivity. Therefore, people who are taking celery seeds need to take a certain amount of precaution when they go out into the sun. Anyone who is suffering from kidney-related issues should also be cautious and speak to their doctor if they wish to take celery seeds.

While consuming celery seeds, users should consume food items that are rich in potassium. This is because the celery seed acts as a very strong diuretic and can hence result in the depletion of the body's supply of potassium. People who take diuretics such as HCTZ or blood thinners such as Plavix or Warfarin should not consume celery seeds unless their doctor has told them to do so.

Side effects of celery seeds could include an upset stomach or a minor amount of diarrhoea. In case you start experiencing these symptoms, you should stop consuming celery seeds.

Dosage

Normally, a dosage of 1 capsule of 500 mg should be sufficient. You can find celery seeds to be available in the form of tablets, essential oil, extract, and either dried or fresh. Any of the available forms can be used. All you have to do is follow the indicated directions that are given on the commercial preparation labels. In the case of celery seed tablets or capsules, two capsules can be consumed two times a day with water. However, take care that you take them after your meals.

The extract can be consumed thrice daily with a ½ or ¼ teaspoon dosage. You can consume this during mealtimes with either juice or water.

Whole seeds can be used in tea. You can take one teaspoon of these crushed seeds, put it in a cup consisting of boiling water, and then make tea in it. This tea with crushed celery seeds can be consumed as much as three times a day.

b) Devil's Claw

When it comes to the pain and symptoms that are associated with gout, the herb called the Devil's Claw is very useful and often recommended for the effective treatment of the condition. The herb is also sometimes referred to as the grapple plant or the wood spider. It is a South African native plant and it is often used for medicinal purposes in the region. This tradition has been going on for a long time. While the whole plant is very beneficial for many reasons, the tuberous roots of the plant are often used in the reduction of fever, for regulating the stomach, and in taking care of the symptoms that are associated with arthritis.

Devil's claw is also great at enriching the body with many of the essential nutrients that it requires. The herb is great at providing the body with minerals such as silicon, sodium, selenium, manganese, magnesium, iron, and calcium. Apart from these, it is also rich in proteins as well as vitamins A and C. Devil's Claw is also a great cleanser of the blood and the bodily systems. It can help to remove the toxins and impurities from the body. This in turn makes the person feel a lot healthier. The healthy feeling that this herb brings in can be especially beneficial for people who are suffering from gout.

Despite the fact that the Devil's Claw is so rich in nutritional content, the real reason why they are so powerful for gout is because of the chemicals called iridoids that are contained within them. These compounds have great anti-inflammatory properties and they are also used to treat the excessive amounts of pain caused by gout attacks.

Devil's claw can also act as a great digestive stimulant since it can aid in the proper digestion of proteins that are consumed. The improper protein digestion can after all lead to a bad case of gout and can cause a flare up to happen.

These two amazing properties of this herb make it extremely popular when it comes to the treatment of gout. Many people have also stated that it can have a tremendous impact on their overall condition.

There are many ways that devil's claw is used. If you are purchasing the herb commercially, then you should follow the instructions on the cover with care or talk to a medical practitioner regarding the dosage that you should be taking. Taking devil's claw in solid form will be ideal since that way you will be able to tell how much you are consuming. If you however choose to consume the liquid form of the herb, then you should be careful and measure the exact amount that you are consuming. The best way to measure is to use either a measuring spoon or a dropper. Some of the mixtures can also be used to make tea.

Devil's claw is also available in the form of creams and lotions that can be applied on the areas of the body that are swollen or inflamed. However, be sure that you do not end up using this herb in more than a single form since there is always a risk of an overdose. If you wish to take this herb in more than a single form, then you need to speak to your doctor before doing so. This will help clarify any risks associated with the product in case of using it in more than one form or accidentally over-consuming it.

There are a few things that you should keep in mind before you decide to consume this herb. It is always a good idea to speak to your doctor about it. They will be able to guide you in the best possible manner. If you are a patient of diabetes, suffer from chronic or recurrent stomach ulcers or issues, or get low or high blood pressure on occasions, then you should avoid it. Care should also be taken if you are on medications that are used to treat the above-mentioned conditions. Always know that you should purchase this herb from a reliable and trustworthy source so that you can be sure that the product is pure and has not been contaminated in any form. Devil's claw should also be avoided in case you want to become pregnant, are already pregnant, or are breast-feeding.

Dosage

In case you want to use this herb to treat gout and its related symptoms, then you should take the following dosage:

- Take 1 capsule of 500 mg on a daily basis
- In case you are taking dried powdered root, then you should take a dosage of 1 to 2 g thrice daily
- In case of a tincture, you should take 4 to 5 ml on a daily basis
- In case you are taking dry solid extract, then take 400 mg thrice a day on a daily basis

Either one of these can be taken on instances of gout attacks.

9. Other Herbs Great For Gout

Arnica
This herb has been extensively used in many of the medical fields including herbal, allopathic, and homeopathic medicine. It has also been an extensive part of the American and European medical histories for a long time. In Europe, people have been

using Arnica in order to cure and soothe aches and pains. The red Indians in America have made use of this herb along with its tincture to soothe any bruises and aches and also to treat any wounds. The Germans made use of Arnica to make healing ointments and creams. In the field of homeopathy, Arnica is a very important herbal medicine that is most commonly used.

Researchers have also pinpointed to the fact that this herb consists of two substances that have anti-inflammatory and analgesic properties. These two substances are known as dihydrohelenalin and helenalin. People who would consider making use of Arnica should be sure to always apply it externally and never ingest it internally. It could be poisonous if ingested. Some of the patients who use Arnica might also suffer from certain allergic reactions such as those on the skin. When that happens, the herb should be discontinued.

Benefits of Arnica

- As an ointment, Arnica can help cure a lot of issues such as inflammations from insect bites, swelling due to fractures, rheumatism, or any wounds, aches and bruises.
- In homeopathy, Arnica is used for easing muscle-related soreness, conditions related to extreme exertion and trauma, as well as wounds.
- Arnica can also be taken in the conditions of shock and the resultant distress.

The best part about using Arnica externally is that it has no side effects, as it is a completely natural product. The results achieved are also amazing since the herb heals from the core and doesn't just focus on the related symptoms.

Cayenne Pepper

Cayenne pepper is available in many parts of the world since it is grown worldwide. The first time humans made use of cayenne pepper was in Latin America. Apart from being great for seasoning food, it also has amazing healing properties.

It is great for treating bloating cramps, stomach pain, or any problems related to the circulatory or the gastrointestinal system.

Healing Properties

Cayenne pepper contains amazing healing properties that are especially great and useful for the gastrointestinal tract system. Cayenne can also be used in case a person is suffering from pain as a result of rheumatism or arthritis.

An active compound in cayenne peppers by the name of capsaicin is used for the treatment of fibromyalgia and is great for curing aches in the joints and muscles. This component is also very strong and is highly effective in the treatment of itching, discomfort, or pain. It is also proven that this compound helps to increase the body's ability to release neurotransmitters that help in reducing pain. Cayenne can also act as an excellent antioxidant.

In many of the studies that were conducted, Cayenne pepper was shown to be highly effective for treating migraine pain. This is one of the reasons why Cayenne is prepared in such a way that it can be applied within the nostrils.

Cayenne consists of substances that match the properties of aspirin. These substances are known as salicylates, and they assist in warming the body by increasing blood circulation and dilating the small capillaries. Cayenne can also be used to block the nerve endings in an attempt at reducing pain. It is even great at stemming bleeding from an open wound.

Weight Control

Many elements that are found in Cayenne pepper have been known to stimulate body heat production. This way, the body's metabolism speeds up and hence stimulates the production of norepinephrine and epinephrine. Both of these are known to suppress the appetite when they are combined.

Blood Sugar Levels

Cayenne pepper helps in bringing down the blood sugar levels in a natural manner. However, in case a person is hypoglycemic, they will have to avoid taking Cayenne pepper completely.

Blood Clots

Cayenne pepper plays an important role in keeping the blood thin so that it flows well and does not contribute to any clotting.

Arthritis

When an individual consumes Cayenne pepper on a regular basis, it helps in blocking the nerve growth factor supply that helps in stimulating a hormone called substance P. This substance assists in transmitting pain signals experienced in the body towards the brain. When nerve growth factor is blocked, it helps in diminishing the pain from arthritis.

Cayenne also helps in boosting endorphin production. Endorphin is a natural painkiller that the body produces.

Side Effects

It is extremely safe to consume Cayeene. However, a burning sensation might be felt when it is used for the first time.

Chapter 5: Highlights Of Current Research

The role that uric acid plays in gout is pretty much understood by everyone. Because of this, there are many medications widely available nowadays that help to ease gout attacks and reduce the severity and risk of any future attacks. With this level of understanding of the disease, gout is also one of the forms of arthritis that can easily be controlled. However, despite this fact, researchers are still trying to study the disease further so that they can continue helping people who suffer from the disease and maybe one day even prevent this disease from arising completely. Some of the areas where a comprehensive gout research has been happening include:

Current Treatments

There have been various refinements in the current treatment of gout. Although there are a lot of medications that are already available for the treatment of gout, the doctors are still trying to figure out which types of treatments and at which dosages are these treatments the most effective. A lot of recent studies that have been conducted show a comparison of how effective the various types of NSAIDs are with respect to the treatment of inflammation and pain that result from gout. In addition, the optimal dosages for the various other types of treatments for the control and prevention of any attacks have also been looked into.

Evaluation Of New Therapies

So many different and new types of therapies have been showing a lot of progress and promise in many of the new studies. These therapies include biologic agents that help in the blockage of tumour necrosis factor, which is a chemical that is thought to play a major role when it comes to gout-related inflammation.

The Role Of Different Foods

While we have proof that certain types of foods can worsen the condition of gout, there are still other types of food that also aid in the prevention of gout. One of the studies conducted by scientists found out that if you consume more low fat dairy products, then men would be able to reduce their risk of gout by as much as half. The reason for such an effect is still not known. There has been another study that shows that vitamin C has certain effects on uric acid. These effects may be beneficial in managing and treating the disease along with all the effects that are linked to the production of uric acid.

Approaches For New Treatment

Many scientists have been studying the various types of cells that have an effect on chronic and acute joint inflammations and how they contribute towards it. The research goals are to basically understand in a better manner how the urate crystals manage neutrophils, which are white blood cells, how the bone cells and the urate crystals interact with each other in such a way that could result in weak bone lesions in people who might be suffering from chronic gout, and how the immune system could be affected by urate crystals, thus resulting in chronic gout. These scientists hope that with increased understanding on the subject they will have more innovative ways to treat the disease.

The Effect Of Environmental Factors And Genetics On Hyperuricemia

Many researchers have been studying the various populations where gout might be prevalent so as to see how environmental factors and genes may have an effect on the uric acid levels within the blood, which can crystallize within the joints and thus lead to gout.

These new research and current approaches can have a significant impact on how gout will be treated in the future.

Chapter 6: Complications Due To Gout

When a person has gout, a number of complications can arise as a result of it. The most common of these complications is perhaps the amount of damage that the affected joint will have to endure. This damage can ultimately lead to pain that lasts a long time, joints that become deformed, or even disability in the long run. Apart from this, there are also other complications such as the formation of kidney stones, eye problems, and tophi, i.e. small lumps that form underneath the skin.

Gout attacks can be severe and extremely painful, and if the chronic ones are not treated in a timely manner they can cause severe problems later on in life. Gout complications can exist in two categories. The first is where the joints are affected and the second is where the joints are not affected. Here are detailed examples of complications that arise due to gout:

1. Kidney Disease Or Damage

Kidneys can be damaged if the uric acid crystals are not filtered out of your body and are thus allowed to collect within them. The National Kidney Foundation has stated that many people who are affected with gout also suffer from kidney disease. Kidney disease, if left untreated, can ultimately result in kidney failure.

However, it is not sure whether kidney disease that existed prior to a person getting gout has any affect on the increase in the uric acid levels within the body. Some experts think that prior kidney disease might be a cause of gout to occur in the first place.

2. Kidney Stones

Kidney stones can develop within the body due to the increase in the levels of uric acid crystals in the urinary tract. High levels of uric acid can also result in the formation of calcium stones. About 10 to 25% of people are known to develop kidney stones as a result of having gout. Some of the kidney stones might also cause an interference with the urine flow, thereby causing pain when the urine is passed. Some people with kidney stones also feel that they have to urinate more often. Kidney stones can infect the urinary tract.

If a kidney stone is small, then it can pass through the urinary system and out of the body in a very natural manner. However, plenty of water should be consumed, as water will aid in the flushing out of these stones. Medication may also be prescribed so that your urine can become less acidic. The less acidic the urine, the more it can help in dissolving the stones that may be found in the system. If kidney stones are present in high concentrations, then they can even cause interference in the normal functioning of the kidneys.

The likelihood of such kidney stone formation can considerably be reduced if you reduce the risk factors that contribute towards gout. Such factors can be reduced with simple lifestyle and dietary changes. Kidney stones should never be left untreated since they can lead to chronic kidney disease. The stones can easily be treated with the increased intake of fluids, having the right medications, changing the diet that you consume to make it more relevant, or having a procedure to remove the stones out of the system.

3. Tophi

Sodium urate crystals are the cause of tophi. They tend to form in tissues located inside and outside of the joint. When these crystals start building up underneath the skin, small yellow or white lumps may form that are called subcutaneous tophi. While tophi are painless in most cases, they can be formed in places that are awkward, for instance, around the toes or at the end of the fingers. In most cases, tophi are developed years after the initial attack. However, some cases have also been recorded where tophi has been developed even before an acute gout attack was experienced.

Tophi will usually occur in the heels, forearms, elbows, toes, and knees. However, they can also occur in other parts of the body, even in the vocal chords or the spinal canal. The conditions of the latter are extremely rare.

If tophi are found underneath the skin, then they will also be present within the joint bones and cartilage. When tophi occur, gout might have progressed at a severe level, and this should be enough reason to start treatment if you have not already done so. The tophi can be prevented from getting bigger or even reduced completely in size once the uric acid crystals in the system are lowered and dissolved completely. In some cases, tophi can be inflamed and as a result a discharge can be produced that consists of a mixture of urate crystals and pus. The urate crystals are white in color and often like toothpaste.

If you happen to have tophi that is painful or large or both, then this tophi will hinder you from performing everyday tasks, such as getting dressed or preparing food for yourself. Therefore, if you have the condition, then talk to a doctor about how you can make your life easier, and follow a regimen that will help in reducing tophi. If your tophi are extremely painful and large, then you might have to undergo a surgical operation to get them removed.

Tophi normally cause pain when you have a gout attack. This is when they will become swollen and inflamed. If you allow tophi to continue growing, they might even erode the surrounding tissues and skin of your joints, thereby causing severe damage and even joint destruction in extreme cases.

4. Joint Damage And Deformity

The build-up of urate crystals and the formation of tophi within the bones and cartilage of the joints can ultimately lead to permanent damage or deformity of the joints. If you do not make a conscious effort to significantly reduce the levels of uric acid in order to treat gout, then the attacks that happen in the future will become all the more prolonged and frequent. This will also increase the chances of your joints becoming permanently damaged. If this case becomes extremely serious, then a surgery

47

may also be needed in order to replace or repair the joint that has been damaged. This is because the damage can be such that it can cause misalignment of the joints and even immobility.

The chronic form of the disease would involve the severe symptoms to be on a much lower level. However, the condition would also persist within the joints for a longer duration of time. When such a chronic stage is allowed to stay for such a long time, joint damage will almost be inevitable. The damage and deformity will be permanent in the bones and joints in such conditions.

5. Heart Disease

There has been a high association of gout with cardiovascular disease such as a stroke or a heart attack in many of the studies. It has been stated that people who are affected by coronary heart disease, heart failure or high blood pressure have increased chances of developing gout. This is because the high uric acid levels can result in a higher risk of a person dying from a cardiovascular disease.

In one of the studies it has been reported that the complications that arise as a result of gout can even result in unhealthy levels of lipid and cholesterol. Another study showed that if a person is affected by gout they could increase the risk of getting a heart attack, even if they have had no history of such heart-related problems.

When people are affected by high levels of uric acid within their body, there is an increased chance of them dying as a result of cardiovascular disease. However, it is still not clear as to whether the condition of hyperuricemia itself has any direct association with the increased risk of death as a result of cardiovascular disease. Therefore, scientists and researchers are not yet sure whether the treatment of gout will actually have an impact on reducing the occurrence of cardiovascular disease in individuals suffering from gout or not. However, new studies have been created in order to find out whether cardiovascular conditions in individuals suffering from gout can actually get better or not with the help of medications that aid in lowering the uric acid levels within the body.

6. Psychological Effects

Apart from the physical impact and discomfort resulting from gout, the disease can also impact patients psychologically by having a significant effect on their daily home and work life, as well as their mood and mental health. Due to the severe pain experienced from the condition, getting around even short distances can be quite difficult, making the patient unable to do even the simplest tasks themselves. This can also lead to mental problems such as anxiety and depression. Talking to your doctor can help you achieve solutions to the problem and make your daily life a lot easier, especially when you are suffering from an attack. Your doctor will also be able to help you when you are feeling anxious or depressed.

7. Disruption Of Lifestyle

The complications that arise due to gout can cause extreme pain and even disability. This can also hinder proper sleep. The most common time for gout attacks to happen is at night when you are fast asleep. Therefore, when these attacks happen, they wake you up, after which it can be extremely difficult for you to fall back asleep. The lack of sleep or sleep interruptions due to constant waking up in the middle of the night can lead to problems such as stress, mood swings, and fatigue.

Gout attacks can also hinder you from performing your everyday tasks such as household chores, walking, and going to work, since the attacks can be quite painful. If these gout attacks were to repeat on a frequent basis, then this can even lead to the damage of the joints, which can sometimes even be permanent. When gout is not treated properly and in a timely manner, it can lead to a chronic disorder, which can be extremely painful and can even disable a person completely. Not treating gout at all could also lead to the destruction of the bones and the cartilage, thereby causing loss of motion and even joint deformities that might be permanent in most cases.

Most people who have experienced gout have stated that the pain resulting from the disease is one of the worst that they have ever had to experience. The flare-ups can make walking around, playing sports, and even putting on shoes quite troublesome. Tophi that result from gout are one of the causes of joint deformities and damage. These can grow quite big and thus destroy the surrounding cartilage and bone. If tophi exist in the spine (a condition that is quite rare), then the damage sustained can be significant. This damage would include compression. With the complete destruction of the joints and bones, a person will be bedridden and unable to walk.

8. Other Conditions

If gout is allowed to persist in the long-term, the uric acid crystals will ultimately form in many of the tissues of the body, and lead to a lot of damage. The persistence of gout can also cause the following conditions to happen:

- Dry eye syndrome
- Although rare, gout can also cause uric acid accumulation within the lungs, where it can cause significant problems
- Cataracts, which is also the clouding of the eye lens, hence impairing vision
- Spinal stenosis

9. Outlook In The Long Run And Reducing The Risk

If you want to ensure a good outlook in the long run and have the capability of managing your condition in a better manner, then you need to make sure to follow any advice that your doctor gives you. Medications can significantly contribute towards lowering the levels of uric acid within the body. With lowered levels of uric acid, you will not only be reducing future gout attacks significantly, but will also lower the risks of other complications such as kidney stones and joint deformities.

If your gout has been diagnosed early on, then you will likely face much fewer troubles and can lead a normal live. However, with gout that has advanced significantly, you would have to make sure to lower the levels of your uric acid within the body so that you can remove tophi and improve the function of your joints. Relevant changes in your diet and lifestyle, along with the medications for gout, can also be of great help in dealing with the symptoms of the disease. These changes can also aid in the reduction of the severity of any future attack of the disease and can help you to lead a much better life.

Chapter 7: Certain Questions That Can Arise From Gout

How Does Gout Affect The Body?

Gout is known to affect the joints that are located in the arms, legs, and feet. As the time passes, the flare-ups as a result of gout can increase in their frequency, the number of joints affected, as well as pain. Since gout is known to be a progressive disease, it can eventually cause the joints to stop functioning and make you immobile, especially if it is left untreated. In the extreme cases of the disease, deformity can also arise.

20% of people who were affected by gout have also reported having been faced with kidney stones in the process. A gout attack will cause a sharp pain the body that will only grow worse with time. A person with gout might also experience redness, inflammation, swelling, and pain in the joint. This mostly occurs in the joint of the big toe. The symptoms do however go away on a gradual basis. While gout has three stages, many people never have to experience the last stage with proper care and treatment.

If I have only suffered from one attack, would I have to get my uric acid levels checked and reduced?

Gout medicine or that related to making sure your uric acid levels remain low is not needed if you have experienced gout once. The breakdown of purines within our bodies is what causes the levels of uric acid to rise. These purines are present in bodily tissues and also come from certain food items that are high in purines. Our bodies are normally equipped with the mechanism of keeping the levels of uric acid from increasing. However, when a stage called hyperurcemia is reached, then the levels of uric acid might become a problem, since they become too much for the body to remove effectively. Not all people who have hyperuricemia however will be affected by gout. A few reasons why you would have to take the medicine for lowering your levels of uric acid include:

- Suffering from gout attacks that would not respond as efficiently to anti-inflammatory medicine
- Having 2 or more gout attacks within a year
- Having developed kidney stones due to high uric acid levels within the urine
- Having developed polyarticular gout, i.e. gout that affects more than one joint at a particular time
- Tophi, i.e. the uric acid crystal clumps that are highly visible on the skin, typically near the outer ear and joints. They are also extremely hard.

If need be, the uric acid levels can be lowered by the following methods:

- Indulging in regular exercises and keeping your body weight at healthy levels
- Not over-consuming calories
- Limiting beverages and sugary drinks
- Avoiding processed and red meat
- Avoiding consuming alcohol or drinking in limitation
- Consuming coffee with less sugar if required, since coffee helps to lower the levels of uric acid
- Vitamin C can also be useful in some people for lowering the levels of uric acid

If I develop Gout, when does it become necessary to call the doctor?

If you happen to develop joints that are tender, warm, red, or swollen, or if you happen to suffer from great pain in one of the joints, then it might be necessary to call or go see your doctor immediately.

Seeing a doctor is important in such situations, even if you feel that the pain has stopped or reduced considerably. This is because the build-up of uric acid that caused the attack from gout in the first place might still be present around your joints and can cause some greater damage later on if you do not take the required action. You doctor can then give you medicines that can help in the reversal or prevention of the build-up of uric acid.

You may see one of the following individuals for your treatment and diagnosis of gout:

- Family medicine doctor
- Internist
- Nurse practitioner
- Orthopaedist
- Physician assistant
- Rheumatologist

Why is it that gout often first appears on the foot or feet?
The uric acid crystals will always more likely settle on the parts of the body that are much cooler than the rest. The toes and feet are one such region of the body where the temperature is much lower than other portions of the body. Therefore, the initial attacks will most likely happen in either one or both of your big toes.

Do children have the tendency to develop gout?
The chances of children developing gout are extremely rare. If a child were to develop gout, it would usually be due to the fact that they inherited the disease from their parents, and this disease then caused an effect on their levels of uric acid and the potential of the kidneys to cleanse the system of these excessive levels of uric acid. If a child has certain cancers like leukaemia, that can also increase the risk of a child developing gout.

Why is gout more common in men as opposed to women?
The primary form of gout is much more common in men as opposed to women due to the change that puberty brings in men. This change results in the kidneys pulling back more of the uric acid into the blood. While the levels of urate rise considerably in both the genders after they hit puberty, the increase is more considerable in men. However, a rare condition that is normally

inherited can lead to an over-production of purines within the body. This over-production of purines can result in an increase in the risk of the development of primary gout in both the genders as well as young people and children.

If there is primary gout, then is there secondary gout as well?
Yes, there is secondary gout as well, and this secondary gout can develop in either of the two genders, irrespective of how old they are. The symptoms of secondary gout are the same as that of hypeuricaemia, or high urate levels within the blood. However, this case involves other causes of gout such as:

- A disorder, like fructose intolerance, methyl malonic aciduria, or glycogen storage disease
- A metabolic disorder
- Poisoning due to lead
- Cell destruction as a result of physical damage or chemotherapy
- Prescription of drugs, like diuretics (which help in the lowering of urate levels within the blood), as well as pyrazinamide (which is used in the case of tuberculosis and is known to interfere with the uric acid excretion by the kidneys

If gout runs in the family, then is everyone with a family history of gout most likely to be affected by it?
While it is not yet known to what extent lifestyle factors or those related to a person's genes play a role in affecting the person's gout condition, there may be a strong link. In most cases, a person develops gout due to the fact that their levels of urate present within the blood have been high for too long, and this is due to the capacity of the kidneys exceeding overtime and hence the crystals being deposited. The future generations of men with a family history of gout might not suffer from the disease provided they keep other risk factors such as high blood pressure, a diet rich in purines, and obesity extremely low.

You should also note that people who have certain rare disorders will most likely have a family history of gout.

Can gout affect women before they reach menopause?

Women who have not reached menopause are, in most cases, well protected against the occurrence of gout. This is due to the fact that the normal levels of oestrogen, a female sex hormone, help in excreting uric acid via the kidneys. After menopause however, the oestrogen levels fall drastically, unless a woman is provided with a Hormone Replacement Treatment. This means that there is very little chance of a woman of a younger age to develop gout, and if they do, they should visit a doctor immediately. The doctor will then run some tests for a metabolic disorder as opposed to assuming that the gout resulted from improper excretion of uric acid.

If a person develops gout after starting drugs to control high blood pressure, will they suffer from attacks as well?

Gout is becoming highly common in women who are middle-aged or older. It is especially common in those women who have been prescribed drugs that are diuretics, i.e. water tablets. While women excrete uric acid from their bodies in a much better manner compared to men, the drugs for high blood pressure, especially those that are diuretics, can decrease the overall ability of the body to excrete the uric acid. Attacks related to acute gout are not very common in older women. In a situation where an older woman develops lumps on her body as a result of gout, the disease is referred to as topha-ceous gout. While some of the tophi may be large, the others may be found in the skeleton, and this can cause some serious damage that can be very evident in x-ray pictures.

Can gout unexpectedly arise from a serious illness?

While such a situation can arise, it is highly uncommon. Uric acid is formed when cells die at the end of their life cycles, and release purines as a result. These purines pass in the blood system of individuals. Therefore, a wasting that might occur after some major operation, serious accident, or cancer and related therapies can result in hyperuricaemia, then gout, and ultimately even kidney failure if not treated in a timely manner.

If you look at cancer alone, the growth and death of the cells happen at a much faster pace than in normal situations. For instance, when cancer cells end up traveling from one location to another, they end up destroying nearby cells, and they themselves multiply further. Thus, the rate at which urate is being produced far exceeds the kidney capacity for excretion. This can result in hyperuricaemia and then gout as a result. This is considered to be a secondary gout form since it happens as a result of another disease.

The treatment of cancer might involve chemotherapy or radiotherapy with drugs or x-rays respectively. This results in a large amount of tumour cells being killed off, and due to this, a lot of purines are released into the system. Such a release could result in a tremendous increase in the levels of uric acid within the blood as well as urine, which could give rise to secondary gout. The increase in the levels of uric acid could even result in acute kidney damage due to the blockage of collecting ducts situated within the kidneys. Tophi could also appear in such situations. To reduce such a risk, many of the cancer specialists have started recommending the use of the drug allopurinol during the time that cancer therapy is progressing. The dose of allopurinol however needs to be carefully decided since xanthine in allopurinol can cause the formation of stones, and this formation could result in acute renal failure. Some cancer specialists might even inject an enzyme called uricase that would help in the removal of uric acid from the systems of people undergoing therapy.

Can animals develop gout?
Animals can very likely develop gout. Birds, for instance, excrete highly concentrated uric acid. This can be witnessed by the white portion in their droppings. A chicken strain that has been inbred, and that has a urate excretion deficiency can get lumps on its feet and legs due to the deposits of uric acid. They become disabled as a result of this. Also, lizards and snakes produce uric acid as an end product of their metabolism and breakdown of nitrogen.

Paleontologists also have gathered information from fossil bones that dinosaurs most likely suffered from gout.

Higher apes, certain dog varieties, and humans are the only mammals who have significant uric acid levels within their blood. While Dalmatians excrete uric acid from their bodies efficiently, they are still prone to developing uric acid stones within their kidneys. Dogs can however be treated very easily by limiting the amount of purines they consume in their diet, by making sure the urine is less acidic so that more uric acid can become soluble within the urine, and by giving allopurinol so as to slow down the conversion of purines to uric acid.

Is it possible to develop gout even with normal plasma urate levels?

Yes, there is also the possibility that an individual develops gout even with normal plasma urate levels. Right before or during a gout attack, sodium urate would suddenly transfer into the joints for the formation of crystals. This transfer would deplete the urate levels from the blood. The result would be the plasma urate falling to the range that is considered to be normal. However, once this attack passes, the plasma urate levels within the blood would increase again.

Is it possible that people do not develop symptoms of gout despite having high urate levels in their blood?

Yes, this is a likely situation and it is called hyperuricaemia without any symptoms of gout. The situation can occur in people who have renal failure. However, one thing that people should know is that the higher the urate concentration within the blood, the greater the chance will be that crystals will be formed within the joint, thereby resulting in gout. When an individual's kidneys are damaged in any way, they may reduce their chances of developing gout since the uric acid will then be excreted through the gut, thereby resulting in reduced chances of a person suffering from a gout attack.

Why would the body convert the excess amounts of uric acid into unpleasant crystals that are needle-like?

While sugar and common salt form crystals that are cubic, sodium urate will form crystals that are sharp and long and have a distinctive pattern to them when seen under a microscope and in polarized light. The pain resulting from gout is not due to the shape of these crystals, however. Rather, it is due to the chemical attacks resulting from the immune cells when they encounter the sodium urate crystals. This causes swelling and heat around and within the joints.

How do cherries assist in reducing the attacks?

Cherries are rich in vitamin A, vitamin C, and fibre. Many studies show that the levels of uric acid within the body can decrease by as much as 50% if you consistently consume vitamin C. Cherries can also assist in controlling the inflammation of the joints as a result of gout. This inflammation is the primary reason for incurring so much pain in people who suffer from gout. Cherries are also extremely low in calories and are high in antioxidants. Such properties along with the anti-inflammatory agents within cherries can assist in reducing the risk of heart disease.

Apart from this, cherries also help in fighting against aging, cancers, and many other types of diseases, illnesses, and conditions including depression. When it comes to gout and its relationship with cherries, there are several studies that have been conducted. A 2003 study that was conducted on ten healthy women showed that when they consumed two servings of cherries, they had a 15% drop in their uric acid levels. Another study was conducted in 2006 on 18 adults who were completely healthy. In the study, these adults consumed 280 grams of cherries everyday for a month. The results concluded that they benefitted from a huge reduction of immune cell activity and inflammation-related substances within their blood.

Another major study was conducted for 1 year on 633 patients who had gout. The results concluded that people who had gout and consumed sufficient cherries or a cherry-based extract for a consecutive two days reduced their possibility of having another gout attack by as much as 35%. When patients started eating more cherries, i.e. three servings in each of the two days, then they reduced their risk of having another gout attack by as much as 50%. With a consumption of more than three servings, the patients decreased their likelihood of another gout attack by as much as 75%, especially when the consumption of cherries was in combination with the medicine allopurinol.

A person who has gout can consume cherries in a lot of varieties and forms. For instance, it has been thought that consuming cherries raw, canned, cooked, frozen, black, sweet, or in a pill or tart form can all be beneficial for a gout sufferer. Cherries in a juiced, fresh, or dried form are all equally good, so a patient with gout does not have to worry. If you eat 25 cherries, then you can benefit 10 times more than taking other pain relievers such as aspirin. It has been suggested that you consume around 30 to 40 cherries after every four hours in case you suffer from a gout attack. The same amount should be consumed on a daily basis too, regardless if a person is suffering from a gout attack or not, since it is a great food item to counter gout attacks in the future. The best part about cherries is that it has less fructose compared to pineapples, grapes, bananas, apples, and oranges. If you consume 60 cherries or more in one day would you risk a negative effect of fructose from cherries in the case of gout. However, having 12 to 25 cherries everyday would be fine.

Tart cherries are known to be more effective against gout and other forms of arthritis as well as the in the treatment and prevention of gout-related painful conditions when compared to sweet cherries. They have higher amounts of anthocyanins and phenolics, and are also lower in sugar than sweet cherries.

What do I do about my feet if I develop gout?
When a person develops gout, they can have a significant amount of symptoms that develop as a result. These symptoms are particularly visible in the lower leg and joints in the foot where pain can even arise as a result. It is a good idea to take some kind

of medication such as the NSAID pain relievers to help with the swelling and the pain. Prescription medications can also be taken to manage the gout symptoms in a much better manner. If you want to effectively deal with the pain in your feet, then you may do so by keeping your feet as dry and clean as possible, positioning your legs in a lifted position and in a comfortable manner, and wearing shoes that are comfortable.

Is gout much different from other arthritis forms?

Gout is very different from the other arthritis forms that exist. This is because gout is caused by the uric acid crystals after their levels increase in the body. With excessive levels, these crystals collect and build up around the joints and sometimes inside of them as well. While gout may be a progressive disease, it is nothing like rheumatoid arthritis that tends to attack the organs and bones of the body.

In addition, the word arthritis indicates an inflammation within the joint. Gout is an acute variety of this arthritis. The acute attacks resulting from gout are also normally accompanied by flu-like symptoms, an upset stomach, or fever.

If a person has gout, can they risk developing other forms of arthritis later on in life?

The simple answer to this question is that yes, they can risk developing other forms of arthritis later on in life despite having gout. These other forms of arthritis include rheumatoid arthritis and osteoarthritis. In fact, the damage that is caused to the toe joints in gouty arthritis can result in osteoarthritis later on in life. Therefore, it is highly important that you keep such damage to joints to a minimum so that you do not have to suffer through added troubles later on.

Apart from the regular drugs that you might be taking for gout, you should also pay attention to eating a healthy diet, exercising sensibly, and maintaining a healthy body weight. These will help to prevent many degenerative diseases that are now becoming so common in many people, especially older ones.

Are there medications that can increase my risk of getting gout?

Medications that are used for treating hypertension known as thiazide diuretics can increase the levels of uric acid within the blood significantly. If aspirin is taken in larger doses, then this can also significantly reduce the effect that drugs taken for the disease itself can have on the body. You should therefore have a word with your doctor and let them know about any medications that you might already be taking so as to avoid any potential complications.

Can gout result in heart attacks?

While cardiovascular disease and gout are closely tied together, there is no direct association between them. Many diseases such as diabetes, high cholesterol, and high blood pressure can also result in both cardiovascular disease and gout.

Can gout result in the development of osteoarthritis?

Gout can very much result in the development of osteoarthritis. This is especially due to the chronic inflammation as a result of gout that can add on to the degenerative changes that are caused in the joints, thereby leading to osteoarthritis.

Do medications for gout have any side effects?

Medications that are given for any kind of gout attacks, be it long term or short term can have a few or even significant side effects in some cases. For instance, the medications that are used to change the levels of uric acid can lead to a gout attack or even worsen a current attack. This especially happens with fluctuating uric acid levels. This is a major reason as to why attempting to lower the levels of uric acid is postponed until the acute and painful attacks are gone.

NSAIDs are certain medications for gout that can have side effects such as corticosteroids and stomach irritation, especially during a short-term use in the case of a gout attack. The drug can also cause stomach irritation, insomnia, and issues related to keeping the blood sugar levels under strict control in people who have diabetes. Another drug that is used in the case of gout attacks is called Colchicine or Colcrys, which can result in gastrointestinal side effects such as diarrhoea. Since there are potential side effects for such drugs it is the best idea to consult your doctor before you start taking any one of them for your gout. Your doctor will also be able to help you by guiding you with what medication will be best suited for you considering your conditions.

What happens when gout medications do not have any effect on me?

Certain patients feel that taking gout medications has had no impact on their condition and they still feel the same. However, it is best to consult your doctor under such conditions because you might be in need of some new medications.

Are there certain medications that can interfere with the ones I am taking for gout?

There most certainly are certain medications that can cause an interference with the ones that you are taking for gout. For instance, allopurinol or Zyloprim is a drug that decreases your levels of uric acid within the body. There might be a certain danger attached to taking this drug with other medications. Therefore, it s always a good idea to consult your doctor before you start any over the counter drugs or supplements with the drugs that you have been taking for gout.

Some of the diuretics are also known to worsen the condition of gout. Therefore, these diuretics should not be taken with your gout medications and instead be replaced with other medications that do not cause any harm. Certain medications that are required to be taken for some cancer treatment or after getting an organ transplant can also have a bad reaction with gout medications and on-going therapy. Aspirin should not be taken since even a low dosage of the drug can lead to high levels of uric acid and the retention of uric acid. However, if you take aspirin in a high dose, it can actually lead to the levels of uric acid being lowered. However, never take this without prior approval of your doctor since it could have a bad side effect.

Is pseudogout and gout the same thing?

While pseudogout is like gout, there is one very important difference between the two; that is gout is caused by the formation of uric acid crystals within the joints whereas pseudogout is a result of a salt known as calcium pyrophosphate dehydrate, or shortly known as CPPD. Pseudogout is also sometimes known as a CPPD disease.

Pseudogout normally results in acute arthritis in one of the joints. In most cases of pseudogout, the joint of the knee will be affected and the attacks of this form of gout will normally last for a few weeks, whether they are treated or not.

Some of the symptoms that result from pseudogout however are very much like the symptoms associated with gout such as the onset of swelling, pain, and heat in the joint that has been affected. Pseudogout would normally result from excessive calcium in the blood that could result from the overconsumption of vitamin D or the overworking of the parathyroid gland. It could also occur as a result of the disease called haemochromatosis. In this disease, a lot of iron gets deposited in organs such as the liver. This condition has no link with excretion through kidneys or foods that are rich in purines.

Some of the treatment aspects of pseudogout are very much similar to those of gout. These include removal of the fluid from the joint that has been affected, a corticosteroid injection, or the use of anti-inflammatory drugs. Attacks would usually subside after a few days. Some of the fluid may be removed by the doctor for the confirmation of the diagnosis, since the calcium pyrophosphate dehydrate crystals can easily be distinguished from those of sodium urate under a microscope with polarizing light.

Is there such a thing as a stubborn gout misdiagnosis?

Many times, people who have been diagnosed with gout complain that despite not indulging in purine rich foods or consuming alcoholic beverages, and being on their prescribed medications, their gout symptoms are worsening. There could be two reasons for such a problem:

The first reason is that you might not actually have gout but another form of arthritis that is often confused with the condition of gout. If your doctor did not conduct a fluid test on you where they are required to extract fluid from the joints that are affected to check for the presence of urate crystal, then you might want to visit your doctor again. You might just have another form of arthritis such as:

- Reactive arthritis: this is a form of arthritis that results from an infection that has happened in another part of the body like the genitourinary tract of the gastrointestinal tract
- Pseudogout: this is where calcium crystals get deposited within and around the joint instead of uric acid crystals
- Infectious arthritis: this happens as a result of an infection that occurs inside the joint
- Psoriatic arthritis: this happens in four to six per cent of individuals who happen to have psoriasis, which is a skin condition

If someone experiences a more chronic or later stage of arthritis, then this stage can also be confused with osteoarthritis or rheumatoid arthritis.

The second reason why your issue with gout might not be mellowing down or being treated effectively is that the medications you are on might not be taken in a sufficient dosage. A study that was conducted showed that around 50 per cent of the patients who were taking the standard dosage of allopurinol, a drug that reduced the amount of uric acid within the body, were not reaching the maximum target of lowering the levels of serum urate within their bodies. If you have recently retested for gout and the results came to be positive, then you might want to consult your doctor about increasing the dosage of your drugs.

Can gout be caused as a result of fasting?

Fasting can definitely result in gout. Normally, fasting involves a person not consuming food or water for a designated amount of time. When a person does not drink water for a considerable amount of time, they can get dehydrated. This dehydration can result in the increase in the levels of uric acid within the body.

If a person suffers from severe pain in the gut and develops gout right after, was the pain in the gut the cause of gout?

Gout can arise as a result of an acute illness. A severe pain the gut due to any reason could also trigger gout. For instance, if the pain in your gut was the result of food poisoning, then this food poisoning or even dehydration could have resulted in gout.

What should I know about whey protein supplements if I suffer from gout?

Bodybuilders and athletes very popularly take whey protein supplements since these products are known to help build and maintain muscle, especially after intense sessions of exercising where your amino acids can get entirely consumed and hence depleted.

Whilst whey proteins are not directly linked with the disease, these proteins can cause an excessive burden on the kidneys where they have to work extra hard to clear out and excrete these products from the system, especially when the kidneys are already finding it hard to excrete out the uric acid from the body. A person with gout should consider that their kidneys are already finding it difficult to rid the body of the uric acid that can excessively build up within the body. And whey proteins are not all that easy to excrete out.

If you still wish to use whey proteins, it is a good idea to consult your doctor before doing so. Your doctor will be well aware of the advantages and disadvantages of doing so since they will know all about the health of your kidneys along with the medications that you are talking to help with your gout treatment.

They will also be able to evaluate the status of your muscles in a much better manner.

Will consuming folic acid lower the levels of uric acid?

A few of the studies that have been conducted recently have been studying how folic acid affects the levels of uric acid within the body. Scientists have primarily been studying the effects of folic acid on the excretion and production of uric acid. These studies have concluded that there is no effect of folic acid on the excretion and production of uric acid. Therefore, increasing the consumption of folic acid in the case of gout cannot be recommended since it does not seem to have any effect on the levels of uric acid within the body. However, the potential effect of folic acid on gout can be studied further in order to determine whether there is any effect or not.

Are solid lumps on the back of the hand and on top of the ear connected to gout in any way?

The lumps that are formed by urate crystals are called tophus. Apart from settling within the joints, the lumps can occur on the elbow, heel, toes, back of the hand or outer ear. In most cases, the lumps will be seen on people with long-standing or chronic cases of gout. However, in some cases, when a tophus develops on the skin, it could signify the first gout symptom. Sometimes, this tophus might even burst through the skin and reveal a chalky deposit. The doctor will be able to recognize this as urate crystals by taking a sample of this chalky deposit and testing it in under polarized light with the help of a microscope.

Why do certain people develop gout despite never over-eating or drinking heavily?

While beer and foods rich in purines may be major contributing factors to a gout attack, these are definitely not the only causes for a gout attack. Heavy exercise, various medicines, stress, and dehydration can also be the contributing factors to gout.

If you happen to be a young and healthy man, there is an increased possibility of you having a mild metabolic disorder form. This can cause an increase in the levels of uric acid within your blood, thereby further contributing towards triggering a gout attack.

If you suffer from a gout attack, then be sure that you limit the intake of foods containing purines. In case your blood urate levels still do not drop, then you should contact your doctor immediately.

Why does a gout attack happen so suddenly, especially considering that the crystals keep accumulating for so many years?

Hyperuricaemia, which is the high urate levels within the blood, can occur for many years. However, the symptoms of this may not occur early on. A number of different situations or events can cause a trigger of a gout attack. These situations or events include a surgical operation, an injury, drinking, or binge eating. Some people also happen to be extremely sensitive to certain food items. Therefore, it is best to avoid them.

Why do painful gout attacks come and go?

The crystals of sodium urate have the ability to re-dissolve if or when the concentration of these crystals within the plasma falls and when the excess amounts of these crystals are excreted through kidneys.

However, this concentration can increase again with more of the sodium urate being deposited. This can cause a repeat in the symptoms.

Is there any connection between kidney stones and gout?

Since uric acid is not very soluble, it can be deposited in the form of stones or as crystal accumulations within the kidneys of certain people, especially if they have acidic urine. If these stones are allowed to remain within the kidneys, an infection risk could develop significantly, either within the kidney or other portions within the urinary tract. If the stone is to pass through the ureter, i.e. the tube that passes from the kidney to the bladder, but is hindered due to its size, it could result in the obstruction of urine flow and severe pain. This can lead to an increased amount of pressure within the collecting system and hence the damage in the kidneys as a result.

If a person develops diabetes and their kidneys become damaged, can this lead to gout?

Arterial disease is highly common in people who have Type 2 diabetes, which normally develops in adults, especially the adults who suffer from high blood pressure or are overweight. In most cases, this runs in the family. If your kidney circulation becomes affected, then the efficiency of your filtration process will become affected as well. This would mean that in the case of a high risk of gout, either as a result of increased uric acid production or having a diet rich in purines, a gout attack could occur. You should definitely follow a proper exercise and diet plan to help you lead a healthy life in case you have diabetes, and also maintain a diet that is low in purines. Speak to your doctors so that they can keep the urate levels within your plasma under strict control.

Can kidneys suffer permanent damage as a result of gout, or can their function improve if drugs are used and a proper diet plan is followed?

People who have gout may suffer from mild kidney damage. However, this does not mean that their kidneys will suffer from permanent damage or will fail eventually. While there may be people who have had kidney disease as a result of hyperuricaemia as well as secondary gout, the conditions of these people have been far different from the people who have ordinary gout, and therefore only suffer from mild kidney damage.

People with a high amount of hyperuricaemia may have their uric acid crystals deposited into their kidneys. Such a condition is more common in people who have inherited genes that are linked to an X chromosome gene. The first symptoms that occur as a result of these conditions appear mostly in childhood.

Is it okay to call your GP during your first gout attack or should your drive to the hospital instead?

It is extremely important that you get the required treatment as soon as possible when your joints become painful, hot, and inflamed. While the diagnosis may lead to gout, it is essential that you get the condition tested to check for an infectious arthritis. The treatments for the two types will be quite different and hence you need to be sure that you have gout.

In case a GP cannot see a person immediately, it is a good idea to visit the hospital.

Are there any symptoms one should look out for that act as an early gout attack warning?

Many people have reported a fever as well as a general feeling of being unwell when they were about to have a gout attack. This feeling of being unwell is probably a result of the effect produced by a chemical substance that is released into the blood due to a response by the body's immune system. Some people have also had a gout attack right after suffering from an upset stomach. They might have also experienced very yellow urine, a common sign of dehydration. Therefore, it is extremely essential that you keep yourself hydrated, especially if you have had too much alcohol.

Do winters bring about more gout attacks?

If a person suffers from more gout attacks during the winters, then this could be the result of stress caused by viral or bacterial infection, consuming more spirits or beer on New Year or Christmas, or eating more, especially comfort food. However, the summer season brings about more possibilities of dehydration from intense exercise or hot weather. This can also result in a gout attack.

In case of another gout attack, is it important to call a GP or visit the hospital again?

If everything is going according to plan, the treatment for gout will most likely be satisfactory. Most GPs will be familiar with the treatment of this disease. Therefore, if a person suffers from another gout attack, calling their GP will be sufficient. In rare cases however, a person will require specialized treatment, in which case they might have to visit the hospital again. The specialist that they should visit in this case is a consultant rheumatologist.

Why does gout affect some of the joints and not others, especially the big toe?

In the areas of the body that are far away from the heart, tiny blood vessels, i.e. capillaries pass through, in which blood flow is more restricted and as a result the temperature is lower. Such conditions encourage more of the sodium urate to form crystals and get deposited within the joints. For this reason, the joints that are located in the extremes of the body, such as the feet and even the hand at times, are more likely to be affected with gout attacks. Usually, the first attack would involve one of the joints to be affected. This is known as monoarticular gout. In the case where more than one joint is affected, the condition is known as polyarticular gout.

When someone suffers from a painful joint, should they rest or get on with their work?

When you are suffering from excruciating pain in your joint, especially when it comes to the joint of your foot, then you should always rest and not force yourself into any other activity, no matter how important it is. Indulge yourself in a warm bath or put a warm pack over your foot. However, be sure that the water is not too hot that you end up burning your skin and tissue.

Cold packs are also effective when it comes to reducing the pain that occurs as a result of gout. It is also easier to grab a cold ice pack compared to a hot water bottle. In case you are thinking of using a walking stick, be sure that it is of a correct length and is fully able to support your body.

Once the pain disappears, how should one get around in the best possible manner?

It is best that the individual wears comfortable and soft shoes so that the swollen joints are well accommodated. The shoes should also be easy to wear, such as those that are trainer style shoes or soft slip-ons. Bedroom slippers are also a great choice. Search for shoes that have a rigid sole or a sole that has been specifically designed to accommodate the shock coming from contact.

In case of temporary swelling or permanent deformity, visit a podiatrist who will be able to help you out by relieving pressure with the help of padding, reducing corn sizes, providing the necessary support in the shoes, or giving you advice with respect to what shoes you are supposed to wear. Shoes can also be made wider so as to accommodate swollen joints.

Will a person's feet be deformed permanently even after the excess amounts of uric acid have been removed from the joints?

This will highly depend on the amount of deformity that has arisen. While the pain and swelling will most likely be there when urate crystals are deposited within the joints, the inflammation will most likely be resolved on its own once all of the urate crystals are removed from the body. The deformity in the feet usually occurs when urate crystals are deposited in the form of clumps within the foot tissues located outside of the joints. This will most likely distort the shape of the feet. In the case of the formation of tophi in the bones, an even further deformity can arise. Such a deformity can cause a lot of problems to an individual and even make it hard for them to walk around. In some cases, the tophi can even burst through the foot's skin, and since uric acid discourages or comes in the way of healing, the skin through which bursting took place can become highly infected. When such an incident happens, one should seek immediate assistance and guidance from a professional doctor or a GP.

With proper treatment, the size of tophi can gradually reduce, and the smaller tophi can disappear completely.

If gout attacks happen early in the morning and a person's feet often remain cold as a result of poor circulation, is it okay for them to wear socks for keeping warm?

If a person's feet feel cold during the night, this could be the result of narrowing arteries. Narrow arteries could in turn be linked to diabetes or smoking. Therefore, you should definitely consider taking care of your diet and reducing the amount of cigarettes you consume. Socks may actually be beneficial for keeping you warm and making sure the urate is prevented from turning into the crystallized form within the joints of the toes. Consider buying a duvet if you do not already have one, since it will keep you warmer compared to blankets or sheets. The weight will also be less on your feet in this case.

If the last gout attacks experienced by a person were a few years ago, will an attack happen again if the person stops taking the drugs prescribed to them?

There will always be a risk if you decide to stop taking the drugs that you were on for gout. The risks include the urate levels in your plasma increasing and as a result an attack occurring. However, you might want to consider taking this risk if you prefer not to be on medication for the rest of your life. However, before you undertake such a huge risk, be sure that you have sufficiently changed your lifestyle in terms of stopping drinking, not consuming a diet rich in purines, and losing weight. You should also consult your doctor on whether you can completely stop taking or reduce the amount of prescription drugs that you have been taking. About 10% of people suffer from a gout attack once in their lifetime. In such case, allopurinol will not have an advantage over such lifestyle changes. Other people may experience attacks on a repeated basis. These attacks often become long lasting and frequent as the time passes, and do not go away even with thorough treatment with drugs.

Will gout worsen as the sufferer ages?

Gout does not necessarily worsen as the person ages. All you have to do is be sure that your urate levels in the plasma remain under strict control through the use of medicine. This way, you will remain protected from any possible future attacks within a period of six to twelve months after you have started using drugs to lower your urate levels. In case a person has tophi, it will also eventually become smaller and smaller. Their tendency of producing kidney stones with uric acid will also decrease. Gout should be controlled in a good manner so that it does not bother you as much for the rest of your life. When a person reaches old age, their kidneys somewhat lose their ability to excrete waste products such as uric acid. This however should not have an impact on gout control unless some other factors cause the kidneys to be completely damaged. There are also certain drugs that cause an impact on kidney function such as NSAIDs or diuretics. These can alter the ability of kidneys to handle urate.

What is the connection between blood pressure and gout?
It has been widely known and accepted that hyperuricaemia and high blood pressure are linked together and exist in a person at the same time. Both of these ailments occur in families, and this means that they are both hereditary. Doctors are very much aware that the two conditions will happen together in an individual in most cases, and if one condition exists, then a person should be suspicious about the existence of the other as well. On top of that, people need to remember that drugs that are used to treat one of these conditions will not have any effect on the other condition. Alternatively, diuretics that are used in the case of high blood pressure might just result in an acute gout attack. Blood pressure increase is never good, and if this is not treated in a timely manner, then it could result in a coronary heart disease or even a stroke. Both of these conditions can be prevented if proper and timely treatment is provided. Lifestyle changes might also be necessary. Many of the lifestyle changes that a person makes for taking care of high blood pressure can also be beneficial for gout. This is a reason why your doctor will carefully keep track of your blood pressure when you go to speak to him/her for gout.

If someone recommends glucosamine sulphate in treating immobility and pain for osteoarthritis, will this be beneficial for gout symptoms as well?

Glucosamine sulphate is a compound naturally found in our joint cartilage. This helps our bone surfaces to move against each other in a smooth manner. In the case of gout, if the crystals of sodium urate have caused enough damage to the joint surfaces, then some of this damage might remain even when the crystals have all been removed. The joints might feel stiff as a result. While many doctors are still sceptical about the functioning of this product, there have been many testimonials from people who have been happy with it since it eased their arthritis. While there is no scientific evidence for the benefits of this product against gout, if taken by mouth, it seems completely harmless.

If a person suffers from a gout attack in the feet, can they still exercise?

They can very much exercise their other body parts. For instance, hand weights can be used and pull-ups can be done. If they want to do aerobic exercise, then swimming is always a very good option in the case of gout. This helps to exercise the entire body without putting pressure on the feet. Continuing exercise will definitely help in keeping the person's weight under control.

Should I indulge in walking or running in between the attacks to prevent the crystals being deposited in the joints?

While walking is a great option, running will put a lot of pressure on the joints, especially on the joint of the big toe. This pressure could result in another attack. Cycling is another great exercise that a person can take up, and the best part is that it does not put any pressure on the big toe, which is especially vulnerable in people who have gout. If you cannot cycle outside due to excessive traffic, then you might want to consider investing in an exercise bike, which you can then use at home.

How does a person with gout plan a vacation for themselves, especially when their attacks are unpredictable?

If a person with gout wants to go on a vacation but is worried about an unexpected gout attack, they should use drugs that lower urate levels on a regular basis. This should be sufficient even if you do not make any changes to your current lifestyle, i.e. diet, exercise regimen, and drugs while you are on your vacation. However, be sure that you drink sufficient water so that you do not become dehydrated, eat carefully, and pay special attention to any gastric upsets that may cause vomiting or diarrhoea. In the case of any emergency, you should keep a leaflet with you containing all the information with regards to strong painkillers and regular drugs that you might need. Some of the antibiotics available in Europe would not even need any prescription. However, be sure that you know what you are getting, since certain antibiotics such as ampicillin can cause an interference with drugs that help to lower urate levels in the body.

The worst kind of attack would be the one that happens right before or during your trip. Therefore, be sure to let the airline you are travelling with know that they should keep a special wheelchair for you just in case. They might even provide you with addition leg space in case you suffer from a gout attack during your flight. This special attention will however depend on how much room there is on the flight.

Can paracetamol help with fever or pain in case of a gout attack?

Paracetamol is not a very strong painkiller. However, it benefits the stomach lining by not ulcerating or irritating it. Paracetamol therefore will not help in the cases of gout attacks. You would need stronger and more relevant drugs such as a drug from the family of NSAIDs in case the pain is extremely severe. Another great drug is a COX-2 inhibitor. This type of drug will most likely not cause too much problems for the stomach.

Are there any drug combinations that a person needs to avoid taking when they are using NSAIDs?

When more than one drug is consumed in a single day, these drugs can react together and produce an effect that might be harmful for the person. Such a reaction is known as drug interaction and some people can be highly susceptible to these effects. For instance, NSAIDs might just react with other NSAIDs or aspirin, anti-epilepsy drugs, anti-clotting agents, and lithium to produce harmful effects for the individual. Alcohol is considered to be another drug with very serious results in some of the cases when it is reacted with another drug.

Therefore, be sure that you have a thorough consultation with your doctor in case you are concerned about any side effects of taking two or more drugs together.

Can a person become addicted to the painkillers they are taking for gout and can these drugs lose their effectiveness over time?

Painkillers like NSAIDs and paracetamol will not lead to addiction. They also do not lose their effectiveness overtime, and will continue to work as anti-inflammatory agents or painkillers over the course of time and by taking the same dosage. You can also continue taking repeated courses of these drugs when the requirement occurs.

However, certain drugs such as opiates, including heroin and morphine, can be highly addictive. If these are used on a frequent basis, then higher dosages might be required to have the same effect. Due to this reason, such drugs will not be best suited in the treatment of gout and should not be consumed for other types of treatments either.

However, painkiller abuse is becoming quite common, especially those that are available over the counter. When it comes to this, one should be concerned. Many of the medicines used for day-to-day ailments such as coughs, colds, and headaches, can easily be purchased and can consist of addictive drugs. These include:

- Stimulants like ephedrine hydrochloride, pseudephedrine hydrochloride, or caffeine
- Narcotics like codeine, an opium tincture, or morphine
- Antihistamine sedatives like promethazine hydrochloride or diphenhydramine hydrochloride

Always be sure that you read the label so as to be sure that you are aware of the warning signs before taking any medication. You also need to be aware of the recommended dosage and make sure that you do not take medication for more that three days without prior approval of the medical supervisor. Analgesics overdose can be very harmful and can even have damaging effects to the liver. There is also another danger of becoming addicted to the medication.

If my GP advises me to take anti-inflammatory drugs, how long would I need to take them?

Slowly and gradually, you can cut down on the NSAIDs or colchicines that you have been taking, provided your urate levels in the body are stabilizing and reaching the point where you no longer have to suffer from any gout attacks. However, be sure that you keep some with you in case you have an unexpected gout attack. Have a thorough consultation with your doctor in case of long lasting or frequent gout attacks.

If co-proxamol starts to lose its effect on me, what else can I use?

In most cases, the inflammation as a result of gout can be highly acute. The pain experienced can also be highly severe, so much so that analgesic drugs like co-proxamol would not be able to control the inflammation and pain sufficiently. In these cases, strong anti-inflammatory agents known as NSAIDs should be used in order to control gout attacks. These days, NSAIDs are used in almost all instances of gout attacks apart from when a person is resistant to these medications. In such situations, corticosteroids should work. These medications can be taken orally for about a week or even injected into the joint that has been affected. The injection can be given into the tissue of the muscle from where the blood stream can be accessed. Another great possibility is the adrenocorticotrophic hormone that helps in stimulating the adrenal glands so that they secrete more hydrocortisone. This is injected into the muscle tissue.

Why can I not take steroids for gout that provide instant relief?
Steroids, also known as corticosteroids, are given to patients in the case that NSAIDs do not provide the necessary effect. For instance, gout attacks can often be very serious and cannot be cured by simple NSAIDs. While the occasional use of steroids is perfectly fine, one should not make a habit of them. This is because steroids can have a cumulative side effect on individuals such as osteoporosis and high blood pressure upon repeated use.

Can medication help in treating gout completely?
While there is no scientific evidence to suggest that medicines can alter gout or hyperuricaemia to make it better, you can trust these medications to ease the pain for you, provided you know which medications to take. Apart from medications, there are many other complementary treatment options that can help a person with gout. These complementary treatment options include aromatherapy and homeopathy, and these can be extremely relaxing and soothing for the body. However, there is no alternative to the drug treatments that you have been prescribed. Therefore, keep taking them.

Will the use of stinging nettles help with gout?
Research has been carried out in order to investigate how the application of stinging nettles near the arthritic joint can help with the pain experienced in the joints in a few days. While the stinging nettles can cause some inflammation and pain of their own, they are thought to help out immensely with arthritis such as osteoarthritis. However, there has so far been no study conducted on the effect of stinging nettles on people with gout. However, if an individual is brave enough, they can give it a shot and let everyone know the results.

Is a person not supposed to have caffeine three days prior to getting their uric acid levels measured?

Yes, a person is not supposed to have caffeine three days prior to their test. This is because caffeine in coffee and theobromine and theophylline in tea consist of chemicals that look similar in structure to uric acid. This similarity can interfere with the test results and hinder accuracy. However, tea and coffee are not the only sources of such chemicals. Substances like cold cures, headache pills, Red Bull, and cola can also contain sufficient amounts of caffeine. Similar chemicals can also be found in confectionery, chocolate, and herbal teas. Therefore, be careful with what you take and make sure it does not have the above stated chemicals.

Other things that you should restrict yourself from taking are antibiotics, vitamin tablets, and other herbal remedies or drugs. If you are confused whether you can consume a certain thing or not, you can always talk to your doctor.

Why must urine be collected for 24 hours if someone wants to test their uric acid levels?

This is because uric acid and related components have the tendency to be excreted at different rates in the day. The first urine that will be produced in a day will usually be the one that has the highest concentration. Uric acid excretion throughout the day will highly depend on what you consume and when you consumed it. Therefore, in order to even out all possibilities, a sample of 24 hours is asked for. This sample will consist of every possible excretion that has happened within that period. While the urine sample may seem large enough to you, the contents required by the laboratory for testing might be very minute. If your sample of 24 hours is a small one, then the laboratory might suggest that you increase the intake of your fluids so as to flush out all of the toxins from your body. You should be able to pass two litres of urine at a minimum every day.

Should a person have their uric acid levels checked on a regular basis despite taking drugs that lower urate?

Once the urate levels in your plasma become normal with the help of urate lowering drugs, you will notice a significant decrease in your gout attacks, and you will eventually become free from gout. However, you need to remember to continue taking these drugs in the dosage that has been prescribed to you. This will help in keeping your urate levels in your plasma low unless an unexpected event has occurred in your body to cause an imbalance in your urate excretion and production. For such an unexpected change to occur, it is important that your urate levels are checked on a regular basis so that you can figure out whether to increase your drug dosage at any point in time. For most people who have stable gout, a blood test after a six to twelve month period will be sufficient.

Are home testing kits available for measuring uric acid levels in the body, just like those available for diabetes?

At this moment, home testing for uric acid is not possible. This is because the uric acid test relies on a reaction that you will not be able to effectively measure at home.

If a person has been taking a diuretic called furosemide for a long time for swollen ankles, will they be at a risk of developing gout?

Diuretics are used in helping to remove excess body fluids. They have been widely used in treating diseases like nephritic syndrome and heart failure. One possible side effect of diuretics like furosemide could be to make the kidneys retain urate. The effect of diuretics is so strong that it can result in gout, or make the existing gout condition even stronger. Therefore, if a person is on these diuretics, it is always a good idea to get the urate levels of the blood checked out, especially if that person is developing symptoms that point towards gout. At the same time, the person should also consider leaving the diuretics, especially if the medication is no longer required. If the person's ankles no longer swell up upon stopping furosemide they no longer need the medication.

If I have gout, will I get uric acid kidney stones as well? If so, how can I minimize the risk?

Uric acid kidney stones will form in people whose metabolism, diet, or lifestyle lead to the risk factors stated below:

- A low urine volume
- A highly acidic urine that is connected with excretion of other diet components and exercise
- A high uric acid level in the urine
- A significant fluid loss through perspiration, especially applicable for people undertaking strenuous exercise or living in a hot climate
- A combination of all of the above stated factors

A diet rich in fish, poultry, or meat is not good in this regard since it leads to your urine being more acidic and your uric acid levels to increase. The general rules to follow are to not take a lot of salt in the food that you consume or consume salty snacks and to make sure to be well hydrated. The ideal amount of urine to be passed each day is two litres at the very least. This will help to prevent stone formation, which is made from less soluble components.

Can an individual check the acidity of their urine at home?

While the laboratory that you give your urine sample to will check the acidity of your urine along with other tests that are supposed to be conducted with the sample, you can very well check for the acidity at home as well. All you need to do is carry out a test that is much similar to the litmus paper test that you might have carried out in your chemistry classes at school. All you need is Dipstix papers that are available in all dispensing chemist shops. These will help to give the pH reading in approximation to the level of acidity of your urine.

Why is it okay for me to consume caffeine when it resembles uric acid and is a diuretic?

While it is true that the molecule of caffeine is similar to that of uric acid, its products after breakdown are far more soluble and therefore it is readily excreted via the kidneys. The only way that it will not be readily excreted is when large quantities of caffeine are consumed. Since cola, tea, and coffee are so widely available, cutting them down in your diet will be extremely tough. And since caffeine is a stimulant and a person can easily form a drinking habit out of it, the wise thing to do here is to not consume more than three cups of these drinks in a single day.

Diuretics like concentrated fruit drinks, alcohol, and coffee cause a lot of water to be excreted through the kidneys. This can result in dehydration, even if adequate fluid amounts are consumed. Apart from this, coffee also provides the body with significant quantities of nicotinic acid. This assists the kidneys in retaining urate instead of throwing it out of the body. Therefore, this fact gives another good reason for reducing the consumption of such drinks and consuming more water instead.

Once I start taking allopurinol for gout, can I resume drinking beer?

Beer is one of the main causes of an increase in the urate levels in the plasma. Therefore, one needs to be extremely cautious if they wish to resume drinking their beer. However, if you want to do so, you can wait for your blood urate levels to stabilize so that your gout attacks can stop completely. Once that has happened, you may start consuming small amounts of foods rich in purines and have beer only in strict moderation so that any chance of further attacks can be minimized. However, be very careful as alcohol, especially when consumed on an empty stomach, can have a great effect on the kidneys as it increases urate retention within them.

If I take a little bit more allopurinol during special occasions, can my urate levels be adjusted like the blood sugar levels for diabetics?

The blood urate levels can instantly rise once the purine intake of an individual increases. This especially results from eating rich meals on those special occasions. However, the urate levels would not fluctuate as rapidly or widely as the sugar levels of the blood does. This would also mean that allopurinol would not be acting as rapidly on the urate levels in the blood as insulin would on the blood sugar levels. Therefore, there is no reason for you to be taking additional allopurinol in the case that you overeat at these occasions. Just try not to overdo it or not get into the habit of it.

If I experience a loss of appetite, will that affect the amount of allopurinol I should be taking?

It is highly important that you continue taking the same dose of the drug you are on and that has been prescribed to you, no matter how you are feeling. The drug can be anything from allopurinol to even an uricosuric drug. The same is true even in the case of illnesses such as the flu and a cold. However, you need to drink sufficient amounts of water so that the amount of urine you produce is good enough. Take special care of your water intake when you are feeling feverish. This is the only way through which you will be able to maintain your plasma urate levels at a constant rate. This will ensure that you do not get any gout attacks in the future.

If I don't want to take drugs, then is it okay if I stop taking allopurinol and just try to treat my gout by eating healthily?

There is no doubt that a huge difference to your gout symptoms and general health can be made by consuming less calories, beer, and purines. If you take up certain measures that help in fighting high blood pressure, diabetes, and heart disease, and make an attempt to stay away from salt, sugar, and animal fats, then this can contribute greatly to your overall joint care. While you may be one of the few people who would be able to remain without a gout attack with a simple change in your diet, you should remain vigilant about future gout attacks and take the medication on a regular basis once the attacks start again.

Will allopurinol lose its effect overtime?

No, allopurinol will never lose its effect. However, if the medicine fails to take its proper effect as time passes, then there could be a possible explanation for it. Here are some of the explanations:

- You might not be taking a proper dosage as recommended to you by your doctor. You need to be sure to check the bottle label so that you can be sure that you are still aware of what the correct dosage is. The most common way that the drug fails to take its effect is when the person fails to take the drug according to proper prescription and dosage.
- You may require more allopurinol due to a certain reason, which you may not be aware of. The reason could be anything from the exercise regimen that you are following or the diet that you are eating. In this case, you must check the levels of urate in your plasma to see whether it can be considered as hyperuricaemia or not. If that is the case then you might want to increase your dosage of allopurinol upon the recommendation of your doctor. This will help to ensure that your urate levels fall back to normal levels.
- Another reason for this could be an additional drug like an NSAID or a diuretic or even a kidney disease that is completely unrelated to the condition, which might have caused damage to your kidney's ability for uric acid excretion. Either of the above-mentioned drugs might encourage the retention of uric acid as opposed to their excretion. In these kinds of situations, it might be helpful to start taking a combination of benzbromarone and allopurinol.

If I develop a skin reaction to allopurinol and do not feel all too well after consuming it, should I stop taking allopurinol and take something else instead?

An allergy to anything can easily be caused when the immune system of our body decides to react to that particular thing in a violent or exaggerated way. This reaction will usually result in a rash in most cases. While the rash may be uncomfortable, it will almost rarely be serious. However, in some people, the reaction developed as a result of allopurinol could lead to problems in the kidneys and the liver. These problems can even be life threatening at times. In case allopurinol is causing such issues for you, then you should instantly speak to your doctor and get off the drug. Allergies with allopurinol however are extremely rare and people consume it all around the world without experiencing any negative side effects.

You can tackle allergies with allopurinol by going for one of the following options:

- Substitute sulfinpyrazone or probenecid for allopurinol. Both of these drugs are uricosuric and are well known when it comes to the treatment of gout and hyperuricaemia. However, a little bit of caution needs to be taken with these drugs, especially of you have the tendency of forming kidney stones made from uric acid. The accumulation of these stones could ultimately lead to kidney failure.
- A method exists whereby a person suffering from allopurinol-related allergies is desensitised. The approach is uncertain, tedious, and slow and therefore is not recommended unless the allergic reaction is extremely mild. The approach involves starting with a small dose of the drug and then doubling the dose eventually. This will continue on until the dose that is usually therapeutically provided is achieved. This will bring the whole exercise to an end.

Can women take allopurinol while pregnant or hoping to get pregnant?

In most cases, women who are younger do not develop gout. Therefore, if a woman who is younger has gout she should first get a thorough check-up from her doctor to know why this is so, and if she has a certain metabolic disorder, then whether this disorder has a chance of being inherited by the children or not. For the tests, she might have to provide urine and blood samples so that the GP can send those over to the specialist in order to analyse them thoroughly.

The woman should then decide what her next steps should be. Most doctors would not want to prescribe allopurinol or any uricosuric drugs out of fear that the drugs might have a negative or damaging effect on the development of the baby. While there have been cases previously where healthy babies have been born to mothers who had been taking allopurinol throughout their pregnancy, however, the risk will always be there, especially if there is sufficient damage to the kidneys of the mother.

It is also highly important that pregnant women not take colchicines or herbal remedies that might contain colchicines. This is because these remedies have been proven to cause damage to the baby's development.

Are there any long-term consequences to just relying on anti-inflammatory drugs for gout attacks instead of taking allopurinol?

If your urate levels remain at the normal level, then it should be perfectly fine to not take allopurinol and just rely on anti-inflammatory drugs. However, if your plasma urate levels are high and remain that way, either due to the natural purine over-production or having a diet rich in purines, and you make a decision to not take allopurinol, then you might suffer from successive acute gout attacks. Also, the intervals between these gout attacks will eventually become shorter and shorter. There is also a chance that you suffer from increasingly protracted and severe attacks. As more and more months pass, the urate being deposited in your tissues and around your joints will increase, and these deposits could have a great damaging impact on the adjacent bone. This will then become eroded and result in severe deformities, especially those in the foot. This will cause extreme difficulty in walking. You might have to limp or even rely on a wheelchair or walking stick for walking support. If a person is ready to suffer from all of that then they might as well let go of allopurinol. However, the risk of doing so is huge.

In the case of gout, can white wine be considered better compared to red?

Both the varieties of wine are equal contenders when it comes to the occurrence of a gout attack, considering the two have a similar content of alcohol. Alcohol is known to cause dehydration, especially if consumed without food. Some people have however reported that red wine results in certain issues for them. The reason for this could be a heavy tartrate deposit in the wine that might cause an attack to occur.

Why does a person have to continue watching their diet despite taking the prescribed drugs for gout?

The drugs prescribed to you assist you in keeping the high uric acid levels under strict control. If they are not controlled properly, then they can keep accumulating in the blood and result in an unexpected attack. This therapy should continue on for the rest of your life since only a handful of people can treat their gout-related symptoms with just food. Allopurinol helps in the slowing down of uric acid build-up in the blood. Uricosuric drugs help in the elimination of uric acid as it enters the kidneys. Foods that are rich in purines can greatly affect the levels of uric acid within the blood. This uric acid will eventually form crystals. Therefore, while it makes sense that you should think before you eat, it also makes sense that you take your prescribed drugs and on time.

If your daily prescription of allopurinol is low, or you have been asked to take tablets on alternate days, then this might be indicative of the fact that your kidneys have not been working in an effective and efficient manner. Your doctor will therefore want you to restrict the amount of purine rich foods that you consume and your beer intake. This should help in controlling the amount of purines that you end up consuming so that your allopurinol dosage can remain low for a long time. People who have metabolic gout should not consume a dosage that goes beyond 300 mg since there is always a danger of xanthine accumulation within the kidneys.

If my husband develops gout, then can I prevent my sons from developing the disease?

In a few of the cases of gout, men have inherited the tendency to develop the disease. Therefore, you should definitely be concerned about your sons developing the disease as well. However, you should know that there is a high chance of men developing the disease at middle age and not when they are younger. Encourage your sons to have more fruit or salads and perhaps dishes made out of stir-fry or pasta that consist of less purines or meat. This will also encourage your husband to consume options that are healthier for him in terms of his gout. You must also let your sons know how important it is to eat healthily, what gout is, and general information related to obesity and gout. The information that you give to them should especially come in handy when they are out with their friends since they might binge on foods or drinks that they should essentially avoid, particularly beer. When they are out, there is not much you can do apart from letting them know the benefits of eating healthily before they leave the house. When they are going off to university, they might want to figure out how to cook their own meals so that they do not remain dependent on the meals that are provided to them or eat a lot from outside. You can help tremendously by giving them ideas with respect to meals that are low in purines and fat, and are also easy, economical, and quick to make.

Are gout attacks more frequent when a person is having a busy day without even having time for a tea or lunch break?

When you are suffering from gout, you should definitely not miss out on your meals. This is especially true in the case of fluids as fluids are extremely essential for the help that they provide in the flushing out of the toxins from the body. Hence if urate levels are allowed to accumulate within the body, then this could lead to a gout attack.

Would several small meals throughout the day be better in the case of gout or should a person stick to their regular mealtimes?

It is a lot more sensible if you consume a larger meal during lunchtime so that your body has enough time to excrete the uric acid throughout the day. This might not be possible if you are highly busy at work. Therefore, your arrangements should be executed during the weekends. It is advised to never skip your meals no matter what. A regular routine would be great so that you can eat happily with the other members of your family and not feel left out at the dining table.

Consuming sufficient amounts of fluid is also very important, and this consumption should be spread out equally throughout the day and in the evening. While it may be highly inconvenient to have to urinate at night by getting out of bed, this is still better than having to suffer from a miserable gout attack.

Chapter 8: Important Findings And Recent Information On Gout

Below are some of the very important findings that studies conducted in the past few years have shown. The studies conducted on various group of people have prompted various valuable conclusions and data that can further be used to extract far more information when it comes to the treatment and care of patients with gout. Without a doubt, gout is a very bad disease to have. However, there are steps that people can follow in order to prevent gout completely or make sure people who already have gout do not have to go through any future gout attacks.

People with gout might be at an increased risk of diabetes

The inflammatory arthritis known as gout might cause the risk of type 2 diabetes to increase within individuals, and this especially holds true for women. Many researchers analysed around 35,000 individuals who were suffering from gout within the UK and found out that women who suffered from gout had 71% more chances of developing diabetes than those who did not have gout at all. Men, on the other hand, had a 22% chance. Gout might just be one of the independent factors for causing diabetes aside from the already existing and common factors such as obesity.

The American College of Rheumatology indicated that currently, around 3 million or more Americans suffer from gout, and men are more likely to contract the disease. Diabetes can cause severe damage to the kidneys and can result in heart diseases and even amputations of the limbs. It is important that individuals know about the connection of diabetes with gout so that they can start taking precautions early on. However, while there is a strong association between gout and the increase in the risk of diabetes according to current research, it is not clearly known yet why this is the case, and hence more research will be required to find out the reasons.

Some researchers believe that since gout causes low levels of inflammation that are on-going in nature, and this might cause diabetes. Some of the other risks that both the diseases are known to share include high blood pressure and high cholesterol. These can also result in a person getting diabetes as a result of gout.

Women are more likely to develop diabetes as a result of gout. Researchers said that women with gout are at a 5% chance of developing diabetes whereas men with gout are at a 3% chance. A study conducted also noted that people who had gout went to see their doctor a lot more, took diuretics and steroids on a more frequent basis, drank a lot more alcohol and suffered from far more medical related-issues as opposed to those people who did not suffer from gout. Researchers said that the best possible way to reduce diabetes or gout risk is to control certain factors that contribute to the disease such as cholesterol, weight, and blood pressure. This connection between gout and diabetes raises an integral question for all doctors. The question is whether the people who suffer from gout or diabetes should also get tested for diabetes or gout or not. It is important to think comprehensively when a person suffers from gout or diabetes so as to take steps in order to reduce the chances of contracting or diminishing both the diseases.

Some cases of gout might be diagnosed with the help of CT scans

A new study suggests that the condition of gout that might have been missed in the current and traditional modes of testing the disease, which are also the standard testing procedures, might be detected using CT scans. One of the standard tests involves a needle through which tissue samples or fluid is extracted from the joints that are affected by gout. This sample is then checked to see if it contains uric acid crystals or not. However, the test is not always effective.

Researchers at the Mayo Clinic found that the CT scans that consist of dual energy helped to detect the disease in about one third of the patients who otherwise did not test positively for gout using the needle test. Doctors can make use of CT scanning for patients who might be experiencing symptoms related to gout, yet were not diagnosed positively for the disease. The CT scans helped to pinpoint where the uric acid crystals appeared to be, and then the needle test was conducted on those areas with the help of an ultrasound to check for the presence of uric acid crystals. Many patients even remain undiagnosed for so many years consecutively, and this can actually be harmful for a patient.

However, CT scans should not be the first mode of diagnosis. This is because the standard testing procedures for gout are far more effective in most cases and superior as well. It is important to get the disease tested as soon as possible since it requires medications that are different from those that are required for the treatment of other inflammatory arthritis conditions. A patient can then focus on changing their diet and taking proper drugs so as to minimise or prevent any future attacks from gout or the spreading of the disease to the other joints in the body.

CT scans can really help doctors and researchers understand the disease in a better manner and learn how the disease manifests and where it can occur.

Gout patients should drink enriched skim milk

If a person has gout they should seriously consider consuming enriched skim milk. This is because skim milk might help in reducing the amount of flare-ups that a person with gout experiences, and these flare-ups can be quite painful. A study was conducted on 120 patients who had gone through two or more flare-ups in the duration of the four months. These patients were then divided into three groups, where one group was made to consume enriched skim milk containing glycomacropeptide, the second group was made to consume a milk fat extract of G600, whereas the third group was made to consume lactose powder.

Previous research on the effects of milk showed that people who consumed lesser amounts of dairy products were at a higher chance of developing gout. Earlier research has also indicated towards the trend of a decrease in gout attacks as a result of an increase in the intake of G600 and GMP, i.e. glycomacropeptide.

The milk that was given to each of the groups was consumed once on a daily basis and the flare-ups of each patient were noted to have decreased. Out of the 120 patients that initially came in, only 102 completed the entire duration of three months. Out of these, the group that consumed enriched skim milk had reduced their episodes of flare-ups significantly and more compared to those patients who were present in the other groups. The patients who consumed enriched skim milk were also known to experience major improvements in their levels of uric acid within the urine, tender joints, and the overall pain that they experienced. The study also noted that enriched skim milk had no impact on the weight of individuals, and in no way did it increase the harmful fats in the blood.

This study showed that a person who suffers from gout should drink enriched skim milk to reduce the flare-ups that they experience as a result.

Certain foods might contribute towards gout flare-ups

Seafood, meat and other food items that contain a lot of purines in them are really bad for people with gout and hence should not be consumed. They can result in immediate gout flare-ups or trigger attacks when consumed. However, research has not been able to prove whether they have the tendency to result in immediate attacks or not. Research was conducted on 600 plus patients who had gout. Most of these patients were men who had an average age of 54. These patients were studied for an entire year and during this time the patients suffered from gout attacks around 1,250 times. Most of these attacks were experienced in the toe region. It was recorded that when a person did not experience a gout attack, they consumed about 1.66 grams of purines within a two-day period. However, the individuals who did suffer from a gout attack after these two days consumed about 2.03 grams of purines. Individuals who consumed purines the most were 5 times more likely to be affected by a gout flare-up than those who consumed minimal amounts.

Sources of purines that came from animals such as seafood and meat increased the likelihood of an attack by many times compared to the plant sources of purines such as peas, oatmeal, lentils, mushrooms, spinach, asparagus and beans. Apart from having lower amounts of purines, these plant sources also have a high nutritional value and compounds that help to lower the resistance to insulin. This compounds aids in the control of the disease and can actually be beneficial as a result. Other sources of purine-rich diets include alcohol and yeast. Researchers said that a person who suffers from gout should reduce or completely eliminate the consumption of purines in their daily lives, especially those found in animals. This practice can significantly aid in the reduction of attacks experienced as a result of gout. However, while the study that was conducted showed that there was a link between the increased frequency of attacks and the consumption of purines, there was no proof of a direct relationship for cause and effect.

Sugary beverages and increased gout risk in women

A new study suggested that women who consumed beverages that were rich in fructose such as orange juice and sodas that were sweetened with sugar were at a higher risk of developing gout. The occurrence of gout within the United States has significantly increased. This increase can be noted from the fact that in 1977 there were 16 in 100,000 people who were affected by the condition, and this increased to 42 in 100,000 in the year 1996. The increase related strongly with the consumption of fructose and sodas. Beverages that consist of a lot of fructose can especially cause the levels of uric acid to increase within the blood, and this increase then leads to the condition developing.

The study included data from about 78,906 women who did not suffer from gout when the study started. During the course of 22 years, around 778 women out of the original number developed gout. The study compared women who had less than one soda than contained sweetened sugar within a month with those who had one soda every day. The study concluded that those who barely had the soda were 74% less likely to get gout. However, women who consumed more than one soda a day were at a higher risk by as much as 2.4 times. Apart from this, the researchers also found that those women who had one serving of orange juice every day had a 41% more chance of getting gout as opposed to those who consumed less than a glass a month. Those women who had more than one serving developed a 2.4 times higher risk of developing the disease.

The study also showed that women who consumed the highest levels of fructose had a 62% more chance of developing the disease compared to those women who consumed the least amount. Doctors should know how threatening high levels of fructose can be on individuals, especially if they have gout or are at a risk of developing gout.

A common drug for gout could potentially reduce the risk of early deaths

A new study that was conducted found that a drug that is extensively used in the treatment of gout may help in decreasing the instances of premature deaths in patients who are suffering from gout. Research that has been conducted before indicated high chances of people dying early as a result of gout. The study showed the effects of a drug called allopurinol, i.e. a medication that is most often used in the treatment of patients suffering from gout, and how it might help in decreasing the risks of early deaths.

The background information of this study showed how allopurinol caused fatal reactions in around one in 260 patients the drug was prescribed to. This made doctors a little reluctant in prescribing the medication to patients with gout.

Data from more than 5,900 patients was looked into within the United Kingdom who had been prescribed the drug allopurinol. The researchers then carried out a comparison of this data with a group of patients who were not taking the drug. The results showed that patients who did take allopurinol had an eleven per cent less chance of dying from the disease and other related causes compared to those patients who were not taking the drug at all. The study concluded that the overall picture showed that allopurinol had the potential to reduce the risk of deaths in patients by as much as 19%. The reduction in the risk was very clear during the first year of the study and then the subsequent years that it was tested and followed up on.

The results concluded that by taking the drug allopurinol, patients could significantly reduce their risk of early deaths as well as treat the condition and its resulting effects. The results also indicated that the benefit of an increased survival rate with the drug far outweighs the negatives of potential serious side effects.

While the study talked about an increase in the association between taking allopurinol and significantly reducing the risk of premature deaths, there was no proof of a cause and effect relationship between the two.

New gout studies on toe flare-ups

When it comes to flare-ups as a result of gout, the big toe should not be blamed all the time and is not always the reason for such flare-ups, no matter how many people think it to be true. According to a new study that was conducted, researchers found that people who had a greater chance of suffering from repeated cases and attacks of gout were those who developed their first occurrence of gout in joints other than that of the big toe. These joints included the elbow or the knee.

Researchers indicated that gout results from the build-up of uric acid within the body and is a very painful arthritis form. Medication for gout needs to be taken on a regular basis so as to reduce or prevent the occurrence of the condition. Many patients think that if they experience a flare-up, their medications might not be working. This causes them to stop taking them completely. However, these patients should be aware that if they stop taking medications, their flare-ups could get worse, and hence they need to continue taking them.

Researchers spent thirteen years on average analysing 46 patients with gout. The first attack that these patients experienced was when they were 66 years old on average. Some of the findings of recent studies include:

- Researchers have said that black American patients with lupus who have certain autoantibodies, i.e. autoantibodies that are anti-RNA binding protein, have interferon at much higher levels. This is a protein that results in inflammation. The findings will thus help to explain why black Americans suffer from lupus that is much worse compared to white Americans. The result of this study could help find better treatments and solutions.
- Patients with rheumatoid arthritis greatly increase their frequency of changes in the systolic blood pressure in subsequent health care visits as opposed to people who did not suffer from the disease. This erratic blood pressure had a close association with heart disease. This meant that the doctors were required to pay special attention to the risk of heart disease in such patients.
- Another study that was conducted could potentially assist in finding out the reason why smoking increases the likelihood of getting rheumatoid arthritis. Researchers found out that the people who have a genetic predisposition to some immune response could have their dendritic cells triggered if they smoked. These cells are special immune cells. Rheumatoid arthritis is very different from osteoarthritis. This is because rheumatoid arthritis is an autoimmune disorder involving the attack on the cells by the body itself. Osteoarthritis, on the other hand, is more to do with the wear and tear of the body.

The various risk factors that are associated with gout

Gout results from a uric acid build-up within the body and this build-up then leads to painful and swollen joints. According to the United States National Institute on Aging, below are the several common risk factors that are associated with gout:

- Being male
- Being overweight
- Consuming alcohol
- Not taking care of your diet
- Having a family history of gout
- Having too much uric acid in the blood, a condition which is known as hyperuricemia

Gout might be linked to a gene that has recently been identified by scientists

There was a new genetic analysis that was carried out by researchers in relation to gout. This analysis explained why some people were more likely to be affected by the arthritic condition called gout. The research identified eighteen new genetic mutations that resulted in the increase in the uric acid levels within the blood. This increase was the key cause of a person suffering from a gout attack.

Around 140,000 people were analysed in 70 independent studies that were conducted in the United States, Europe, Australia, and Japan. The data that was gathered from these studies provided comprehensive results. A researcher also indicated that once the genetic components involved in the triggering of the disease in some of the cases are known, it could tremendously help in future studies and the disease and related conditions could better be understood.

Gout has sometimes been referred to as the disease of kings. This is due to the common belief that gout and the respective attacks result due to the intake of rich foods that are normally eaten by rich people, since they are the ones who can afford in on a continuous basis. About two per cent of the entire population suffers from gout, and the condition can be extremely painful.

Researchers are in the hope that if they manage to find any indication of the relationship between the incidence of gout and the role of genetics, then this discovery might pave the way for finding better preventive techniques and treatment for the disease. Some of the therapies and modes of treatment that already exist for gout might cause a few side effects, some of which might be very severe. Therefore, any findings have the potential to find new and better opportunities and treatments for gout, and these new therapies and treatments might improve the condition of the disease for the future generations.

Some new guidelines for better management of gout

It is important to educate patients who suffer from gout with respect to lifestyle choices, treatment options and objectives, as well as the right diet when it comes to recommendations according to some of the new guidelines. These new guidelines would ensure that the doctors and patients are able to fight off the disease in a better and a more effective manner. Gout is a very common inflammatory disease that affects around 4% of adults within the United States. Patients who suffer from gout attacks on a consistent basis will likely decrease their overall quality of life.

The rate at which gout is being diagnosed in people has increased significantly in the past twenty years. Currently, it is affecting as many as 8.3 million people. The development of new guidelines with respect to gout have been funded by the American College of Rheumatology where different researchers gathered together and worked together. These guidelines aim to educate patients so that they can follow methods that are more effective in the prevention and treatment of gout attacks. These guidelines will also provide doctors with the treatment that is recommended for the management of the disease in the long-term.

There is evidence that is indicative of the fact that the rates of gout increase in individuals due to certain factors such as obesity, type 2 diabetes, high blood pressure, metabolic syndrome, and the extensive use of diuretics such as loop and thiazide in order to treat the cardiovascular disease.

These gout guidelines, also known as the Arthritis Care and Research guidelines, have been designed so that people who are affected by the disease can receive better care and attention. The guidelines also indicate some of the best practices in relation to medical evidence that is currently available. The end goal of these guidelines is to educate doctors as well as patients with gout so that they can seek treatment that is most effective and will improve their quality of life and condition in the long-term.

Most Americans might be unaware of the risk factors of gout

A study conducted by the Gout and Uric Acid Education Society Survey showed that the general population is not aware of the risk factors associated with gout, even those who are suffering from gout. This disease is known to affect around 8.3 million individuals in America. A survey that was conducted showed that only about one in 10 Americans were aware that cardiovascular disease was among the risk factors associated with gout. In the same survey, only about one in three of these Americans knew that obesity was also inclusive of the risk factors for gout. Less than one in five individuals were recorded as knowing that kidney disease and diabetes were risk factors of gout.

Men are more likely to be affected with gout as opposed to women. However, women who have reached menopause or those people that have a family history of the condition are also likely to get affected. Gout is growing at a very fast rate within the United States and can occur in any of the joints within the body.

The survey recorded that people who suffered from gout know only a little more than the general population, which was not adequate. The survey results showed that one in 5 sufferers of gout correctly said that cardiovascular disease was one of the risk factors of gout. One in five people also cited diabetes as one of the risk factors associated with gout. One in two individuals indicated correctly that obesity was one of the risk factors associated with gout. Also, the study conducted found that one in five Americans were aware that family history could also be a major risk factor for gout. Two in five patients were aware that the disease can be present in families. Three in five Americans reported accurately that diabetes and heart disease could be present in families.

The results of the survey were quite surprising and they are a cause for major concern, since the occurrence of gout within the United States has tremendously increased in the last 40 years. In addition to this, gout is also linked to other severe diseases and health conditions that are also increasing on a day-to-day basis. While the majority of the Americans are aware that the condition is life-long in nature and will require continuous care, attention and medicinal treatment, they fail to understand how they can increase their or their family's likelihood of getting the disease.

It is important for patients to know that they can manage their disease in a much better manner by following a few modifications in terms of lifestyle and medications. These include some physical activity and changes in the diet. If the disease is not treated in a proper and regular manner, then it could even lead to a person becoming disabled. This also happens when rheumatoid arthritis has reached its advanced stage. However, one in five gout sufferers claimed that they have not taken any steps or measures to make sure that their disease is managed in a better manner. Along with this, about nine in ten sufferers of gout have indicated that the disease has been very interfering with their day-to-day life and makes running their daily errands and going to work much tougher.

The survey conducted also indicated that certain gaps were found in the behaviours, and these gaps could actually help in managing the disease of gout patients in a much better manner. For instance, one in three gout sufferers were successful in making the accurate link between alcohol and the disease. Patients with gout need to understand that they should drink their alcoholic beverages in moderation (if they ever feel the need to), especially taking care about beer since beer is known to contain extremely high levels of purines. Patients who are suffering from gout also need to understand that they should consume the beverages and food that consist of high fructose corn syrup in a highly moderate amount (if they ever feel the need to). This ingredient is found to be in many of the soft drinks, unprepared foods, and sweets.

The results of the survey were positive when it came to how aware the patients were when knowing about the importance of monitoring their uric acid levels. Around nine out of ten patients with gout were recorded to have known that they are required to have their uric acid levels constantly monitored and checked. As opposed to this though, less than half of the patients with gout were known to be aware that their kidney function, cholesterol level, glucose level, blood pressure, and weight also need to be kept in check.

Vitamin C may decrease the likelihood of the occurrence of gout

According to many of the researchers who conducted a study on about 47,000 men over the course of 20 years, the more people consumed vitamin C, the more they reduced their chances of getting gout. During the time that the study was being conducted, 1,300 and more men had developed the disease. When a comparison was being done with those who consumed less than 250 milligrams of vitamin C in a day through various supplements and foods, the men who did consume around 500 to 999 milligrams of vitamin C in a day had a 17% less chance of developing the disease. Men who consumed around 1,000 to 1,499 milligrams of vitamin C had a 34% less likelihood for developing the disease. Men who consumed 1,500 or more milligrams of vitamin C had a 45% lesser chance of developing the disease.

The researchers then calculated that every time the intake of vitamin C was increased by 500 mg, the risk of acquiring gout reduced to 17%. These risks were also similar in the instances of men who were and were not taking the vitamin C supplements. Those men who consumed 1,000 to 1,499 milligrams of vitamin C supplements in one day lowered their risk of getting gout by as much as 34%. This was compared to the men who were not taking these vitamin C supplements. Upon taking 1,500 milligrams of vitamin C supplements on a daily basis, the risk further reduced by about 45%.

The researchers concluded that vitamin C might be playing an important role in reducing the uric acid levels within the body that have the potential to form crystals, which then deposit in the joints and cause excruciating pain. Vitamin C might be helpful in aiding in the reabsorption of this uric acid in the kidneys and then help in increasing the rate at which these kidneys work towards excreting the uric acid and preventing any inflammations. All of these can help in lowering the risk of a person to develop or suffer from gout.

The consumption of vitamin C, if taken according to the study mentioned above, and keeping in mind the upper limit of the vitamin C consumption, might just be a highly useful option in the prevention and treatment of gout. For adults, the upper intake level of this vitamin, which will be tolerable, is less than 2,000 milligrams a day.

While there is no proven link between vitamin C and gout, these studies that have been conducted definitely show some concrete facts related to it and might just help people in the long run. People with gout need to be extremely careful and take whatever steps necessary in order to make sure that they reduce their gout attacks in the future.

Chapter 9: Famous Personalities With Gout

If you have gout then you should know that you are not alone. Some very famous personalities, both past and present, had and have gout. This goes to show that gout can affect just about anyone, and you are not cursed in any way if you are affected by it. All you need is proper care and attention to make sure that you remain free from gout attacks. Without further ado, here are some of the very famous personalities with gout:

Michelangelo the famous painter
Raphael's portrait known as 'The School of Athens' shows Michelangelo, who appears to have gout. His body is weirdly angular in the portrait, and while this might not be concrete enough evidence to suggest that he actually had gout, there are other signs. These include his work habits and living conditions. For instance, he was constantly exposed to lead due to paints and wine glasses that were made from lead. He also ate very little during work and used to work long hours, thereby compromising on his health severely. The artist also had a diary in which he constantly complained about his kidney and bladder related-issues. So, just imagine that Michelangelo painted the Sistine Chapel while he was struggling with the pain associated with gout.

Jared Leto
Jared Leto is famously known for starring in movies like Requiem for a Dream and Fight Club. The 38-year-old actor developed gout in the foot after he gained about 60 pounds for a movie he had to star in called Chapter 27. After he developed the disease, he said that he could not walk long distances and he had to use a wheelchair because of the pain.

David Wells
David Wells was a part of the Toronto Blue Jays and the New York Yankees and was a left hand pitcher. He struggled with the

disease through his entire career of baseball. He indicated how much pain he had to go through and the first time was a complete shock. He actually screamed like a little girl and dropped to the floor instantly when his toe started to hurt really badly.

Maurice Cheeks

Maurice Cheeks is a famous personality who has been really fit his whole life, had played in the National Basketball Association for 15 seasons, but struggled with gout. The first time he struggled with extremely bad gout pain was at the age of 46 and during the time that he was coaching Portland Trail Blazers.

Cheeks was also recorded as saying that it is best to prevent this disease because once you get it, you will never be free from it.

Harry Kewell

Harry Kewell is an Australian soccer player who was 27-years-old the first time he was diagnosed with having gout. At the time, he was playing for the World Cup in 2006. He had to sit out since a gout flare prevented him from playing the game.

Gout caused a lot of pain for him, and he had to use crutches to walk.

King Henry VIII of England

King Henry VIII was known to have gout and suffered from frequent flare-ups and attacks. The king was alive during the years 1491 to 1547. He was overweight and often had a glass of wine or a meat chunk for dinner. All these three aspects are known to increase the risk of gout considerably. The monarch is also one of the reasons that gout was known to be the 'disease of the kings'.

Benjamin Franklin

Benjamin Franklin, a famous 18th century personality, who invented bifocals, discovered electricity, and played a part in founding the United States, suffered from gout.

As a result of gout, Franklin also had to miss a lot of meetings specially held for the purpose of drafting the Declaration of Independence. However, Thomas Jefferson, understanding the condition he was in, sent the documents over to him so that he could make any changes to it that he deemed necessary.

Sir Isaac Newton

Sir Isaac Newton, who was an English physicist and mathematician, suffered from unexpected gout attacks in both of his feet. This happened in the year 1725, two years before he died.

Samuel Johnson

Samuel Johnson, who was a British poet and author, and lived between the years of 1709 to 1784, had gout according to him and his doctors. This diagnosis was done in the beginning of 1775 at the age of 65.

He was known to have communicated to William Bowles in the year 1783 that the gout pains were very severe, though the condition never went beyond the ankles.

Luciano Pavarotti

While pancreatic cancer was what ultimately killed this legendary personality back in 2007, he was also known to have suffered from gout. He also became immensely overweight, which contributed further to the disease.

Jim Belushi

When Jim Belushi, an actor and a comedian, had his very first diagnosis for gout, his ego would not let him seek the treatment that he very much needed. However, he soon had a gout attack during a performance in Reno, and immediately afterwards he went to a rheumatologist. After treatment and taking proper care of himself, Belushi has been free from gout attacks for a consecutive 12 years.

Ansel Adams

While this famous photographer was known to travel a lot on foot through the mountains and the forests while searching for great landscapes to take pictures of, he suffered from both arthritis and gout. These diseases ultimately slowed him and his picture-taking hobby though the later years of his life. He was known to have mentioned that while his spirit was immensely in favour of carrying on, his body was no longer allowing it to happen.

Dick Cheney

Dick Cheney, a former vice president, did not reveal much to the public about his health issues. However, he hinted it to the George Washington University Hospital in 2006 at 3:00 am gave it all away. The trip was made as a result of a drug that he was taking for the treatment of chronic foot ailments. This drug resulted in a side effect. We even got to know that Dick Cheney was on a number of medications for the treatment of gout and heart disease.

Alexander the Great

While Alexander the Great was known to be a great warrior who conquered much of the world that we know of today, he also happened to suffer from gout. While there was not much awareness or treatment available for gout, we do know that he had excruciating gout attacks. He eventually died as a result of malaria.

Queen Anne of England

Queen Anne was known to have suffered from a lot of medical ailments from a young age. She eventually got gout as well. When she was to become queen, she had to be carried to her coronation since she was suffering from a very bad attack of gout during the time. She eventually died in 1714 at the age of 49, and it is thought that the causes of her death were suppressed gout and Erysipelas.

Sir Laurence Olivier

Sir Laurence Olivier was a famous English actor in the 20th century and also received a knighthood. However, the actor suffered from gout flare-ups. The flare-up became especially painful when he was filming for the movie called Bunny Lake is Missing in 1965. This was when Olivier was 58-years-old.

Don Nelson

Don Nelson is a famous athlete and coach who played for the NBA for 14 years and was on the sideline for about 30 years. He also spent some time being the head coach of Golden State Warriors. In 2006, when he had won his 1,200th game, it was reported by the New York Times that he only celebrated with one beer and a cigar. This was because he did not want to aggravate his gout. We all know how consuming alcohol has a direct link to the development of gout and the chances of the person getting more frequent gout attacks in the future.

These personalities are all struggling or have struggled with gout. Some of them very effectively made sure that they took care of the issue properly before it got worse or before they had to suffer from repeated gout attacks. This just goes to show that people who suffer from gout always have an outlet to make sure their disease does not progress. If they take proper measures early on, they can make sure that the disease does not affect them too badly.

Chapter 10: Successful Natural And Home Remedies For Gout

When a person has gout, they might also be affected by many other types of diseases and health problems that are linked to gout such as diabetes, uric acid kidney stones, and hypertension. Therefore, it is important that a person with gout receives proper and adequate treatment. Apart from the necessary medical treatment however, there are also some home remedies and treatments for gout that can easily be followed and can provide relief and quick healing to gout-related attacks and symptoms. Below are the 10 great and effective home remedies in case a person is suffering from gout:

Apple Cider Vinegar

It is already known how great apple cider vinegar is when it comes to the treatment of acidic stomach problems and headaches. However, apart from this, the ingredient is also highly effective when it comes to the treatment of arthritis, particularly gout. Apple cider vinegar is acidic in nature and therefore it is highly effective when it comes to relieving acute pain caused by gout. By adding a little honey to this effective remedy, you can also increase the anti-inflammatory response of the body.

Directions Of Use

Take one glass of water in which you are supposed to mix one teaspoon of unfiltered and raw apple cider vinegar. Drink this mixture twice or thrice a day.

If you think that this remedy is effective on you and is helping you tremendously, then you can also consider increasing the amount of apple cider vinegar you are putting in the glass of water to two tablespoons.

Ginger Root

Ginger is known to have some anti-inflammatory properties that can be very helpful when it comes to relieving inflammation and pain. This ingredient can be used in a lot of ways when it comes to the effective treatment of gout.

Directions And Methods Of Use

- Take equal quantities of turmeric powder, dried ginger root powder, and fenugreek powder, and mix them all together. Take one teaspoon of the mixture and add it to lukewarm water. Consume this mixture two times a day.
- Ginger root can also be added in various cooking recipes and meals that you make for yourself on a daily basis. If you want, you can consume a small amount of raw ginger root on a day-to-day basis.
- Take one half of a teaspoon of ginger root and add this to a cup consisting of boiling water. This should then be mixed well and consumed at least once on a daily basis.
- Lastly, you can make a ginger root paste by adding small amounts of water. This paste can then be applied on any portion of the body or joint that has been affected by gout. Leave this paste on for the next half an hour or so and then take it off. This treatment should be carried out once every day.

Baking Soda

The increase in the levels of uric acid within the body is a great contributor to the occurrence of gout. However, the use of baking soda can greatly help in countering this issue since baking soda helps in lowering the levels of uric acid and hence gives relief to the pain caused by it.

Directions Of Use

Take half a teaspoon of baking soda and then mix it in a glass containing water. Consume this solution up to four times a day. However, take care not to consume more than that. Continue this remedy for two weeks.

Do not consume this mixture more than three times on a daily basis if you happen to be more than 60 years of age. Also, the mixture should not be consumed at all if a person suffers from hypertension.

Lemon Juice

Gout pain can be relieved if the body is alkalised and neutralised of excess amounts of uric acid within the blood stream. This neutralization can be achieved if a person consumes baking soda and fresh lemon juice. Along with the fresh lemon juice, a person affected with gout should also consume other vitamin C rich fruits since vitamin C helps to strengthen the tissues of the body.

Directions And Methods Of Use

- Use half a teaspoon of baking soda and juice from one lemon and then mix these together. Let the mixture rest for a few seconds until there is no more fizzing. After this, put the mixture in a glass full of water and drink it soon afterwards.
- A second option is to take out half a lemon worth of juice in a glass full of water and drink this glass at least three times in a day.

Cherries

You can consume both sour and sweet cherries, and these cherries can assist in the treatment of gout since they consist of antioxidant properties. Cherries also consist of anthocyanins. These can minimize the flare-ups as a result of gout and help in reducing inflammation.

Directions And Methods Of Use

- For patients who are suffering from gout, it is highly recommended that they consume at least 15 to 20 cherries on a daily basis. The results achieved can even be better if they make a start to their daily routine with cherries.
- A second option is to have one glass of black cherry juice on a day-to-day basis. To this glass, you can consider adding some minced garlic cloves.

Epsom Salt

Epsom salt is great when it comes to the treatment of many forms of arthritis, specifically gout. The ingredient consists of a high quantity of magnesium, which also helps in lowering high blood pressure and a person's heart-related condition. Therefore, people suffering from gout and respective attacks should consider putting some Epsom salt in warm water and soaking the parts of the body that have been affected in it. This will help to relieve any pain or muscle aches.

Epsom Salt In Detail

Epsom salts consist of sulphates and magnesium. The magnesium in these salts helps in improving concentration and sleep cycles, as well as relieving stress. It also helps in improving nerve functions and easing the muscles. Magnesium also exists as an electrolyte, and this electrolyte helps in making sure that the enzymes, nerves, and muscles function well and to their full potential. Magnesium also plays an important role in how calcium is used and absorbed by the cells of the body.

Other than this, magnesium is great at preventing high blood pressure, strokes, and heart disease. While magnesium can be obtained from certain food items, the absorption of this magnesium is best through Epsom salts being soaked and then consumed.

Magnesium helps in regulating enzyme activity along with preventing the hardening of arteries and the formation of blood clots. Insulin is made far more effective with the help of magnesium, and this helps in reducing inflammation, cramps, and pain experienced in the body. Magnesium is known to improve the ways in which oxygen is used up by the body.

The sulphates that exist in Epsom salts help in flushing out toxins, the development of the brain, joint proteins, as well as proper absorption of nutrients by the body. They also help in the case of migraines by making them easier to bear or preventing them completely.

Sulphates are also beneficial for brain tissue formation and the detoxification of the body as a whole.

Directions Of Use

- In case you want to take a soothing bath, you can add two cups consisting of Epsom salt into a bathtub full of warm water.
- After this, you can lie in the bathtub and soak your body until the water remains warm.
- Carry this activity out once every week. In case you suffer from severe gout, you can consider carrying this activity out twice or thrice in a week.

Bananas

Bananas are high in potassium content and thus are very effective when it comes to the treatment of gout. The potassium in bananas will assist in converting the crystal form of the uric acid into liquid form so that it will be easier for the body to flush the excess uric acid out with urination. Bananas are also somewhat high in vitamin C, and vitamin C is very efficient when it comes to managing the pain and swelling caused as a result of gout. You should have at least a banana or two every single day.

Directions And Methods Of Use

- Consume one or two bananas on a daily basis. You should very soon notice that your overall condition is improving.
- You can also add a ripe banana into half a cup of yogurt. This should also assist in making sure you do not get affected with diarrheal.

Apples

When people say, 'an apple a day keeps the doctor away', the statement is actually true in most cases. Consuming apples on a daily basis is a very healthy and great habit, and a person should continue doing it, especially if they suffer from gout. Apple juice and apple reserves made at home are also just as effective. No matter what way you consume apples, you should consume them every day.

Directions And Methods Of Use

Experts say that a person should consume one apple after every meal. Apples consist of malic acid, which helps in neutralizing the uric acid within the body and hence helps in providing relief against inflammation and pain as a result of gout. If someone does not like eating raw apples, they can consider having apple juice. Along with apples, you should also have raw carrots on a daily basis.

Grapes

Grapes are alkaline in nature and assist the body in neutralizing the effects of uric acid. They are also great at making sure uric acid build-up can be avoided or it can be easily eliminated from the body. However, in the case of diabetes, proper consultation with a doctor should be taken before bananas or grapes are consumed in the diet.

Directions Of Use

Take a handful of grapes and consume them on a daily basis. In case you suffer from diabetes, you should consult your doctor before eating grapes.

Oranges

Oranges also consist of vitamin C and citric acid that help in the neutralization of uric acid. Consuming orange juice instead of plain oranges will be equally beneficial for your gout and overall health.

Directions Of Use

Consume an orange every day. You can also have a glass of orange juice.

Gooseberry

Gooseberry, also known as Amla, is a great source for obtaining vitamin C. The best aspect about this ingredient is that when you convert it into jelly, jam, or even cook it, it will not lose its nutritional value and vitamin C. Therefore, there is no limitation in the form that you can have this.

Directions Of Use

If you are able to, you should have one gooseberry every morning before you start your day.

Strawberries

Strawberries contain a good amount of vitamin C. Therefore you should have a lot of them throughout the day and gain benefits from them, especially if you have gout.

Directions Of Use

Consume fresh strawberries on a daily basis to help against gout attacks, an increase in uric acid levels within the body, and gout inflammations as a result.

Cucumber

Cucumber is highly beneficial when it comes to gout, mainly because they have such a high amount of water in them. You can also consider consuming cucumber juice for the best hydration possible, and staying well hydrated is highly essential for gout.

Directions Of Use

Try to consume half a cucumber every day with meals or otherwise. You can also juice the cucumber for a wholesome hydration effect.

French Beans

If you consume juice that has been extracted from French beans, you can get relief from the inflammation and pain that is experienced as a result of gout.

Directions Of Use

Consume around half a cup consisting of this juice at least once or twice every day and you can benefit greatly.

Activated Charcoal

Activated charcoal has the potential of absorbing uric acid. Therefore, it is highly effective when it comes to the treatment of gout. People who suffer from gout should bathe with charcoal at least twice or thrice a week.

Directions And Methods Of Use

- Take half a cup of charcoal powder and mix this with some water until the mixture forms a paste. You can then put this mixture in a tub and add some water into it. After this, soak the parts of your body that have been affected with gout for about half an hour or more. This is a great remedy and solution for instances where gout has affected the joint of your big toe or ankle.
- In case any other body parts are affected, you can make some charcoal paste as indicated above and apply this paste on that part of the skin. Leave this paste on for about half an hour and then rinse using lukewarm water.
- You can also consider taking activated charcoal capsules in order to help with your gout inflammation and pain. However, you should consult your doctor before doing so.

Cold Water

If you are suffering from pain and swelling as a result of gout, you can place the affected area of your body in cold water. Take care not to use ice directly on your skin because it can make the condition worse and even cause damage to your skin.

Directions And Methods Of Use

- Take cold water and immerse the area of your body that is swollen or inflamed in it for about 10 to 15 minutes. Repeat this process multiple times throughout the day.
- You can also make use of an ice pack. However, do not place this ice pack directly on the skin as you can risk damaging your skin in the process. Instead, wrap the pack in a towel and then place it on whatever area has been affected. Use this method twice on a daily basis. However, do not use excessive ice packs since that can cause the uric acid to crystallize.

Increasing the intake of water

For people suffering from gout, increasing their overall intake of water can have a positive effect. This is because water helps in flushing out excessive toxins from the body and making the levels of uric acid more dilute.

Directions Of Use

Consume at least 8 to 10 glasses of water in a day.

Increasing the intake of water will also help to counter other diseases that are linked to gout such as kidney-related issues or high blood pressure.

Taking Care Of Diet And Exercise

There are certain foods that are really bad for gout patients and can trigger their symptoms. An example is that of food that are rich in purines. You need to avoid these foods and make sure you consume the healthier choices that are more in sync with gout.

As far as exercising is concerned, patients with gout should make a regular exercise plan for themselves so that they can stay fit and healthy and reduce their chances of further gout attacks.

If you have gout, you should try out these simple home-based and natural remedies to provide you with relief against inflammation and pain. However, keep in mind that no cure will lead to a quick recovery. All it takes is a little bit of determination and time.

Supplements

Diets that are low in purines also consist of low amounts of vitamins B, E, and various other antioxidants. This means that these essential components in the diet will have to be consumed in the form of supplements so that free radicals do not cause damaging effects inside the body. The problems caused by free radicals can actually make the problems as a result of gout more intense and severe. Here are a few supplements that you should be taking if you have gout and thus are on a diet that is low in purines:

a. B complex

You should consume 1 to 3 B complex tablets of 50 mg on a daily basis along with pantothenic acid (B5) comprising of 500 mg. This would be divided into doses so that the body is better able to convert the uric acid within the body in the more harmless compounds.

b. Bromelain

Take 500 mg of bromelain twice a day since it acts as an anti-inflammatory and will help you with gout-related inflammations.

c. Fish Oil

Capsules of fish oil worth 2 grams each should be consumed. You can take them two times in a day every day. This will help reduce the risk of getting inflammation as a result of gout considerably.

d. L-glutamine

L-glutamine is an antacid that should be consumed first thing in the morning when your stomach is still empty. Take 500 mg of this L-glutamine on a daily basis and four times a day.

e. L-glutathione

L-glutathione can also be taken on an empty stomach, and a 500 mg capsule should be taken twice a day, every day. The tablet will assist in increasing the renal cleaning of the excess and harmful uric acid.

f. L-glycine

This supplement also acts like an antacid and 500 mg of this can be consumed on a daily basis and four times in between the meals.

g. L-methionine

L-methionine is great at detoxifying the purines. You can take this on a daily basis, twice a day, and 250 mg worth of it on an empty stomach.

h. *Magnesium Citrate*

This is an antispasmodic that helps to relieve any pain that occurs due to gout. You can take 400 mg capsules three times a day.

i. *Shark Cartilage*

Shark cartilage is great at helping to make any pain experienced as a result of gout disappear within an instant. The supplement will also allow you to consume certain food items that you may have left as a result of your gout within a week without even having to experience any pain that could result in the joint that has been affected. Take three to six capsules every day on a daily basis. After about a month of using this supplement on a continuous basis, you can consider not taking it anymore until you start experiencing the pain-related symptoms again. However, at such a point, you will only require about three to six capsules in one or maybe two weeks. This cycle can be continued later on as well whenever it is required. There is a high possibility of your uric acid levels returning back to normal levels with this supplement. However, even if the levels do not come back to normal, the pain that you have been experiencing will still vanish.

Tissue Salts

In order to prevent the uric acid crystal formation within the body, two 6X Silicea tablets can be taken thrice a day and every day. If you are facing a gout attack, then you can increase your dose of this to 3 tablets on a daily basis as well as equal amounts of Nati. Sulph. and Nat. Phos.

Vitamin C

A high dosage of vitamin C supplements should especially be taken as soon as a gout attack is initiated. A 1,000 mg capsule should ideally be taken after every 1 hour in such instances. You may reduce this to 500-3,000 mg on a daily basis in the case of maintaining your gout attacks.

Vitamin E

Diets that are low in purines also consist of less amounts of vitamin E. Fried foods are especially known to deplete the quantity of vitamin E in them. Therefore, it is essential that you consume vitamin E supplements to counter these low amounts. Deficiency in vitamin E is very harmful in patients with gout since it can lead to uric acid formation in excess amounts. You can start your vitamin E supplementation process by taking 100IU of vitamin E. It should be completely natural. This dosage should slowly and gradually be increased to 600 to 800 IU on a daily basis.

Chapter 11: Chiropractic Treatment And Gout

Visiting a chiropractic treatment facility if you have gout can be a great option. Chiropractors understand the disease quite well and will assist you in making your life with gout much better. In the case of gout, many doctors would usually prescribe various medications, steroids, and anti-inflammatory drugs to treat the condition and keep it under strict control. However, while the approach is great in the short-term, it can lead to many unwanted and negative side effects.

In contrast to this obvious medical treatment for gout, the chiropractic treatment focuses on providing patients with relevant advice related to the lifestyle and dietary changes they should be incorporating. Aside from this, chiropractic treatment also includes chiropractic manipulation to help in dealing with the disease without the use of drugs and helping in reducing pain and swelling significantly. This way, your chiropractor will help you in alleviating gout-related symptoms and they will most likely start the whole procedure by asking questions related to your symptoms and history of the condition. A physical examination will then be performed to test whether a patient really has gout or not.

The Chiropractic Advice

Your chiropractor will most likely tell you that you should limit your intake of alcohol, meat, or any other food item that consists of purines. After this, they will guide you towards what you should be eating to counter the problem. We have seen the sorts of things you should eat in the previous chapter. Couch grass is a special herb that can significantly help in improving the functioning of your kidneys so that your body can efficiently remove the excess amounts of uric acid from the body.

The Chiropractic Manipulations And Adjustments

Apart from the correct diet, chiropractors will also perform certain manipulations and adjustments on the affected parts of your body with the help of ultrasound or heat so that any pain that is experienced in the joints can be relieved. The body will also be brought back into the right alignment this way.

The Chiropractic Exercises

Aside from the adjustments, the patients will be required to perform certain exercises at home. Heat treatments might also be provided.

The best part about chiropractic care is that you will not require any surgery or medication. This means that the technique is completely non-invasive.

Chapter 12: Exercising When You Have Gout

When you have gout, being overweight does not help the situation. In fact, obesity is one of the reasons why people develop gout in the first place. However, a person can lose or maintain a healthy amount of weight with a combination of healthy eating and daily exercise routines. But you need to also take care to choose the exercise regimens that will not impact the affected parts of your body in a negative manner.

When a person has a gout attack or a flare-up, they are required to rest the joints that have been affected. Putting extra pressure on them will just make the situation a lot worse. Therefore, the exercise routines should be carried out in periods where a person is not suffering from an attack or a flare-up.

Another issue that is caused when a person is inactive is that their joints and muscles can become weaker, they could suffer from a bone loss, and they become more inflexible. This happens because gout itself makes a person less likely to walk around and causes them to sit in one place for too long. If the period of such inactivity continues, the subsequent gout symptoms could become even more painful.

1. The Benefits Of Exercising

Exercise can help a person to keep their gout in strict check and encourage the body to heal at a faster pace. If a person with gout indulges in the right kind of exercises, then they can increase their overall energy levels, keep themselves in proper shape, benefit from healthier joints, muscles, and bones, and reduce the pain that they experience considerably.

If a person follows a good exercise regime, then it can also help them to reverse their gout effects considerably. It will also increase their bone density, boost their fitness levels, and build a lot more muscle. Regular exercise automatically starts making a person feel a lot stronger and energetic. In addition, people who have gout must remember that if they wish to reduce their levels of uric acid, then they must combine an effective exercise plan with a healthy diet plan. These people should consult their doctors before they begin any exercise regimen.

2. Note Of Caution

Exercises should be done carefully when a person has gout and the entire plan should be put to rest when a person has a gout attack or a flare-up. This is because continuing exercises in such situations will only make the conditions of the inflamed joints worse. However, a person can continue following their exercise regime once the pain has sufficiently decreased.

Exercising is great at helping to stop excessive uric acid build-up within the body, but it will not rid the body of uric acid completely. In order to achieve that, you will have to incorporate a good diet plan into the regimen as well. It is always a good idea to speak to your doctor or physician before you start any exercise plan.

3. Types Of Exercises For Gout

Here are the different types of exercises that people with gout should do. While none of the patients should exercise while they are suffering from a gout flare-up, it is recommended that these exercise be incorporated into the daily lives of the patient so that their bodies and joints remain flexible and their bodies do not stiffen as a result of lack of movement.

Range Of Motion

Mobility-improving exercises are great at reducing the symptoms of gout. When a person has inflamed joints, they also experience a certain amount of pain with it. With pain, a person is less likely to move around much so that they can avoid being in more pain. However, with decreased motion, weight is gained and stiffness is increased. These two factors can cause worse symptoms of gout to develop. This stiffness will only increase with lesser movement. However, a person can change that by increasing their range of motion with certain exercises.

Strength Training

Strength training in the case of gout will lead to the build-up of more muscle mass. Usually when people have gout they lose their muscle mass as a result of limited range of motion. When the motion is limited because of the pain in the joints, the muscles shrink and relax. This can be bad, especially for people who have gout, as it can lead to a negative impact on the gout symptoms and other body parts as well. The best strength training will be to use lightweights in the beginning and then gradually come towards the heavier weights so that your body can get used to them. This will help in the build-up of muscle mass. Another great exercise is light squats that can be great for the thigh area as it can make this area a lot stronger with muscles that are firmer.

Stretching

When it comes to gout, stretching-related exercises are very beneficial. This is because they help to decrease the uric acid build-up within the body. Stretching exercises also help to increase the range of motion and the flexibility of the joints. Apart from this, a stretching routine before beginning hard-core exercises will help to ensure that your joints and muscles do not get damaged. It will also aid in reducing the after-workout soreness.

Slowly and gradually, a person with gout may increase their exercise levels. This will help to increase their level of endurance. However, it is important to be consistent with the exercise plan in the hope of achieving better results later on.

d. Cardio Exercise

Cardiovascular exercises, also known as aerobic exercises, are great at improving the flow of oxygen throughout the body by increasing the heart rate. These exercises also help to promote weight loss by burning far more calories. However, if you suffer from gout, then you should be very careful before taking part in such exercises and discuss the situation with your doctor first. This is because gout attacks the foot areas such as the big toe first in most cases. Most aerobics exercises are high impact exercises, and they may cause the gout symptoms to become aggravated. If you cannot engage in such exercises for that reason, then you can always think of exercises with a lower impact, such as swimming.

4. Common Questions About Exercising With Gout

Below are some of the common questions that arise when exercising with gout. These will hopefully help to answer some of the greatest concerns that people with gout have when it comes to exercising. Many people even end up forgoing exercise because of their unanswered questions.

What is The Best Time To Exercise?

There is no best time for exercising. It all depends on whenever you are ready. However, keep in mind that skipping your exercise routine, even for a single day, is bad. Of course, you can skip it on the days that you suffer from a gout attack or inflammation. Try exercising when:

- You experience the least amount of stiffness
- The medicines that you are taking are having a prominent effect on you
- You are experiencing the least amount of pain
- You are not feeling too tired

You can consult your doctor about the best possible manner in which you can incorporate the medicines that you are taking with your exercise plan. This might provide you with more assistance and comfort when you start your exercise regime.

How Do I Know If I Have Exercised Too Much?

Different people have different coping mechanisms to different kinds of exercises. This is exactly why you should only pay attention to what your body is trying to tell you as opposed to trying to compete with other people. There is a general guise to the rule and that is: the 'two-hour pain rule'. This rule states that if your body does not calm down or suffers from an unusual or extra amount of pain for about two hours or more after you have finished exercising, then you might have indulged in a little too much for the day. Therefore, this rule will serve as guidance for you the next time you go to exercise. You can then plan the regimen out properly and exercise for a lesser time or less intensely. You may also consult your physiotherapist as to what the best solution for you would be. They will be able to guide you according to your individual situation.

Should I continue exercising if I am in pain?

The very obvious answer to this question is 'no'. As soon as you start experiencing pain that is unusual for you or increasing beyond the level that is normal for you, you should stop. If you continue exercising while in severe pain, you can risk serious injury or even develop gout-related symptoms as a result.

However, a thing to note here is that many people who suffer from gout might experience minor pain no matter if they are exercising or not. This pain should not stop you from exercising. You will only be required to stop your exercising routine if the amount of pain that you experience while doing so is unusually high or beyond what you have experienced before.

5. Safety Tips While Exercising

- Be sure to have a proper talk with your health care professional or doctor before you start off with any exercising program. These people will be able to guide you and tell you what exercises will be the safest for you to do. They will also make sure that you carry out these exercises in a manner that will not result in any kind of injury.
- During the period when you are experiencing a flare or a gout attack, you should not exercise at all and devote all your time to resting. It will only lead to more pain if you do.
- Build up to tougher exercises slowly and gradually, and do not jump to them directly. When you build up on a gradual

basis, you will get used to the tougher exercises in a better manner and build more endurance.

- Start your routine with warm-up exercises so that you do not experience any injuries or pain later on during the exercise.
- Once your session is ending, cool down your muscles and joints with some stretches and gentle movements of the body. This will help in preventing any muscle stiffness or pain when you wake up the next day.

Chapter 12: Other Special Techniques To Manage Gout

1. Massage

While there are not many scientific studies indicating the fact that getting a regular massage significantly helps people with gout, it certainly helps them reduce the tension in their muscles, which then helps them to relax. However, people who have gout should be sure to get a massage from reliable people who have had prior experience in working with people with gout. A little research will help you tremendously in this regard.

2. Aromatherapy

Aromatherapy makes use of scents to make a person feel better and relaxed. Many different types of scents exist and are used for aromatherapy. Each of these scents has their own benefits and uses. Normally, the scents that are used in this type of technique are added to a massage or bath, and are sometimes even diffused or inhaled in a direct manner. More often, the type of method that is used in the application of the scent will be more linked to the purpose of the therapy. For example, if a person is suffering from a cold, then the scents will be inhaled to clear up congestion. In the case of arthritis such as gout, the scents will be massaged on the area that is affected to sooth it.

There are many reasons to make use of aromatherapy. It is beneficial when it comes to relieving any kind of pain, to energise the body, to reduce fatigue and tension in the muscles and body, and to provide general care to the skin. In addition, when such calming scents are inhaled, they work amazingly on the nervous system and the brain.

It is highly important to make use of only the most natural scents when providing aromatherapy. There are many scents that have been derived from flowers, plants, trees, and things in nature. The scents that are derived from artificial sources do not tend to work in most cases, or not at all. Therefore, when artificial scents are used, the process cannot be considered aromatherapy.

The procedure is gaining a lot of importance and is growing really fast due to its effectiveness. Many people make use of aromatherapy in hospitals, clinics, and even at home. It is a completely natural cure for many ailments and pains, including gout, and more and more people are now realizing the effectiveness and importance of such natural cures. These natural cures are also used with the other medicines for a certain ailment to speed up the process of recovery. For instance, aromatherapy is great for patients who want to relieve their pain from gout along with the medicines that they are taking already.

The essential oils used in the treatment and process helps in the stimulation of the sense of smell. Many people have a really strong sense of smell, and odours generally play a very important and powerful role in the way an individual feels. Aromatherapy can help to produce certain hormones that can help in alleviating certain negative symptoms generated by the body.

There have also been various studies conducted in the field showing how inhaling some of the scents can have a stimulating effect on certain regions of the brain. For example, lavender is a special scent that is used to relax the body. Studies show that lavender helps in increasing alpha waves in the back region of the brain that helps in making the body feel completely relaxed and at ease.

Aromatherapy is therefore a tried and tested method for dealing with many kinds of ailments, including gout, and helps the body to feel great in general.

3. Hydrotherapy

Hydrotherapy is a great form of therapy for all those people who are sick and tired of the swelling and pain they experience as a result of gout. While drinking sufficient amounts of water is effective for preventing pain in gout, there are also other ways

131

that water can be made use of for relieving the symptoms of gout, and that way is hydrotherapy.

This method makes use of hot and cold water in the external treatment of gout. It is a great way to relieve any pain that is associated with gout.

Drinking water is beneficial in making sure that a person remains well hydrated. It is also beneficial to keep the joints well lubricated so as to prevent future attacks associated with gout. Drinking water also helps in improving the function of the kidneys. When this is combined with hydrotherapy, the benefits will be seen quicker.

Hydrotherapy can be used in two ways. One is the Standard method and the other is the Contrast method. In the Contrast method, hot and cold compresses are used in the dissolving of urate crystals within the joints when a person experiences an attack. This method helps in reducing the inflammation and pain considerably. These compresses are used alternatively where one of them is used for 3 minutes and the other for 30 seconds. The hot compress is made with the help of a bucket or sink of hot water at 90 or 95 degrees, a bath or a towel, and a heating pad. For the cold compress, ice packs are used. In case of water being used, it should be easily reachable.

Contrast hydrotherapy should not last more than 20 minutes a treatment, and there should be a gap of at least one hour between the treatments, in case more treatments need to be given. The therapy should end by using a cold compress.

In standard hydrotherapy, the entire body needs to be submerged in water. This helps in achieving weightlessness that helps a person to feel relaxed and completely at ease, especially from the joint region. Having to sit in a tub that is full of hot water is considered to be the best form of hydrotherapy. When the bubbling jets massage the body, the blood vessels become dilated. And this helps in improving blood circulation and getting the oxygen to flow in a better manner.

The process also helps in releasing the natural painkillers within the body and is a great way to provide relief to sore joints. The method is used in the treatment and prevention of gout. However, the procedure should only be conducted for a maximum of 20 minutes in a single treatment. Then a certain amount of gap should be given in between treatments. Since the body's weight on the area that has been affected can make the attacks even worse, this hydrotherapy form helps to relieve a portion of the weight of the body in a way that no stress is being given to the affected area. The treatment is therefore spa-like and extremely relaxing and effective in the treatment of gout.

However, all those people who are suffering from gout should consult their doctor before they officially start their treatment for hydrotherapy. You also need to remember that diet is highly important when it comes to gout and this form of treatment is a great choice for all those people suffering from gout.

4. Reflexology

Apart from hydrotherapy, another great alternative treatment for gout is reflexology. This form of treatment has been effective for a lot of gout sufferers.

Reflexology, also called zone therapy, helps in stimulating certain points on the hands, feet, and ears that act as pressure points. When these pressure points are tapped into, the resultant feeling that is experienced throughout the body is very positive. Reflexology thus helps in making a huge difference when it comes to improving the overall health of the body. When it comes to the treatment for gout, reflexology will be administered in the foot region in most cases so that the symptoms associated with gout can be eliminated.

There is a common belief and understanding in the field of reflexology that the foot region has many reflex zones. These zones correspond to certain other energy zones in the body. The theory then suggests that when pressure is applied to these gritty and tight regions of the foot, the energy points within the body will be stimulated. As time passes, reflexology treatment will encourage the body to self-heal as it cures any imbalances in the overall energy of the body.

In reflexology, a qualified professional will pinpoint certain designated areas that exist within the foot and then massage those areas with the help of their hands using no drugs or tools whatsoever. Such treatments help in improving posture and circulation, increase oxygen and nutrients within the cells, help in encouraging pain management, reduce stress, and remove toxins from the body.

When reflexology is used on a person who suffers from gout, the technique assists in restoring balance within the kidneys, i.e. major organs when it comes to uric acid production. This will then ultimately help in reducing uric acid production or break the deposits of uric acid crystals within the joints. These crystals may be present in the joint of the foot and contribute towards gout.

There are no side effects to the treatment in most cases. However, after the treatment is over, some people may have nausea, headaches, or sinus congestion. Reflexologists term this stage as healing crisis and think that it results due to the body removing toxins. Even if these side effects are experienced, they will not last for more than 24 hours.

While reflexology is a great alternative treatment for gout-related symptoms, it should not be used if a person has an active gout case. Therefore, if even the slightest touch hurts, then these people should stay away from massage during the course of that time.

Consult your doctor or physician before you start this treatment, especially if you have high blood pressure, diabetes, cancer, osteoarthritis, or kidney stones apart from gout. If the technique is performed effectively, it can prove to be great for people with gout.

5. Acupuncture

An ancient practice originating from China, acupuncture involves inserting thin and small needles into the skin at specific pressure points on a person's body. This helps to block out pain signals. Studies related to acupuncture and its link with arthritis such as gout show mixed results. However, some people might actually feel that this treatment is beneficial for them when they seek it along with the other treatments like medications.

The treatment makes use of stainless steel and disposable needles and helps in stimulating certain channels that carry energy, thereby relieving illnesses and pain.

Each point that the needle is inserted in is wiped using alcohol first, after which an extremely thin needle will be inserted. These needles will be inserted at various points and at various depths where they will remain from a few minutes to even an hour sometimes. The needles might even be spun in a light manner or heated so that the effects can be increased.

A certain tingling on the skin may be felt during the treatment. In case the treatment becomes uncomfortable, the person performing the procedure should be informed instantly. The reaction of the person during the treatment is also analysed to see whether the procedure is even working or helping the person.

A lot of people suffer from arthritis, especially gout. The disease can really help in providing relief from the symptoms of gout and any related future attacks. In the case of arthritis, the whole body is taken into consideration and not simply the parts that have been affected. When the needles are placed in the treatment for arthritis, they will normally be placed in the arms, toes, shoulders, and legs. Most people who have arthritis do not complain of discomfort when they are receiving this treatment since the needles that are used are extremely thin.

If the patients are scared of needles, then they should be aware that this part would be over as soon as the needles are inserted. The procedure is so calming that some patients even fall asleep while the treatment is going on. The frequency of these treatments will vary according to the requirements of the patient. Typically, acupuncture will last from five to 30 minutes, and occur one or two times in a week. Sometimes, the patients will find relief in just one treatment. However, in the cases of most severe gout, more treatments will be required in order to find relief.

Only go to an accredited and a reliable practitioner when it comes to acupuncture. Also, it is always better to consult your doctor before starting this therapy session.

6. Acupressure

Acupressure is a great alternative treatment and therapy in the case of gout.

While most people might have heard of acupuncture, acupressure might be a relatively new term for them. While it is based on similar principles, it makes use of hands and feet as opposed to needles to apply the designated pressure at the various points on the body. Acupressure is even sometimes called the Shiatsu massage.

The body has a natural healing ability, and acupressure helps to promote and stimulate circulation of the blood so that this self-healing is accomplished. Pressure is applied using the knuckles, feet, and/or hands on certain areas of the surface of the skin so as to release muscular tension. This treatment is great for all of these people who are suffering from inflammatory or stress-related illnesses like gout.

Acupressure helps in unblocking the energy flow within the body, and this ultimately helps the mind and the body to come at a far more natural and balanced state.

When we suffer from an ailment, our bodies often become tense. People who suffer from gout normally suffer from inflammation and pain in the joints, and therefore cannot relax much. Acupressure helps in removing these symptoms and increasing the flow of blood in the body.

Many gout sufferers have gotten relief from the technique in the following ways:

- Tension release
- Improvement in blood circulation
- Increased ability to relax
- Relief from any pain that is felt
- Increased clarity in the mind
- Reduction in the areas that are inflamed
- Reduction in overall stress

While any individual can learn how to apply pressure on their bodies themselves, it is always a great idea to visit a professional. The first feeling that a person gets at the beginning of the treatment is an electrifying jolt. After this, a tingling or a numbness feeling will follow. As time passes, the individuals will experience a decrease in the overall sensitivity towards the treatment. Some gout patients have experienced immediate relief to pain when this treatment was administered on them.

Since this is an alternative therapy, it should be used in conjunction with medications and other treatments for gout. Also, you should always consult your doctor before you begin this treatment.

7. TENS Or Transcutaneous Electrical Nerve Stimulation

A TENS machine applies mild impulses in order to block the pain from any painful area. The use of this machine can be very beneficial to counter pain in the long-term. However, it would not work on all people. Therefore, before you end up buying one, you should talk to your physiotherapist and learn more about it.

8. Mind Techniques

Meditation

Meditation helps in improving the overall health of your body. This is because it helps in reducing your stress and clearing your mind, and also increases your overall efficiency to achieve more in your daily life.

Meditation is known to impact your physical and mental state instantly. All that you require for meditation is a quiet place where you can peacefully sit and meditate without being distracted so that all your stresses can melt away. It also directly helps in reducing the frequency of headaches as well as instances of nervousness and high blood pressure.

Since medication helps you to focus solely on your breathing, it helps to bring the mind and body together. Even some of the scientific studies have helped to prove that meditation helps in decreasing the levels of a stress hormone named cortisol, and also decreases the heart rate and blood pressure. Studies have also shown that through meditation the brain waves in a human being are positively impacted.

Aside from making a person feel more calm and concentrated, meditation also helps in easing any pain that a person is experiencing. This especially holds true for people who suffer from arthritis-related problems and symptoms, including gout. Meditation assists these patients in removing their focus from inflamed joints, thereby helping to reduce their pain as well as decrease depression, fatigue, and frustration that many gout and arthritis sufferers suffer as a result.

Meditation also helps in increasing melatonin production, a hormone that helps you to feel great and improve on your sleep. Since meditation also helps you to enhance your mood by decreasing your stress, it also helps in the muscles to relax and encourages your body to release endorphins.

Meditation is also a very cost-effective way for healing your body in a completely natural manner.

Relaxation

There are certain relaxation techniques such as guided imagery, progressive relaxation of the muscles, and deep breathing exercises that can help in reducing the tension in the muscles and overall stress levels. Such techniques should be practiced on a regular basis. However, you might have to try out a few relaxation methods before you find the one that works out for you in the best possible manner. Certain CDs, books, and recordings can really aid in the learning of relaxation techniques.

Stress Reduction Based On Mindfulness

This is a great program that was developed in the University of Massachusetts. The program helps individuals in becoming more aware of unhelpful or exaggerated thoughts and how they should be responding to such thoughts in the best possible manner.

Distraction

There are certain techniques that help individuals in distracting them from the pain that they might be feeling and helping them cope with it. Such techniques involve reading, exercising, or simply listening to music.

Courses On Self-Management

There are certain courses on self-management that can provide you with the assistance that you need to manage gout in a better manner.

Visit A Psychologist

A simple visit to a psychologist might be able to help you deal with gout. Psychologists can teach you certain mind techniques that might be very beneficial.

Chapter 13: The Cycle Of Pain

Pain, fatigue, depression, and stress are all linked to one another. For instance, people who suffer from anxiety or depression will most likely show more sensitivity towards pain. With more pain comes more depression, stress, and fatigue. Thus the cycle continues. However, there is good news, and this good news is that the cycle of pain can be disrupted by the techniques and strategies used to manage gout.

There are some truly great strategies and techniques apart from the obvious treatments for gout that people have made use of so that their condition can be managed in a much better manner. It is also helpful if the people around the sufferers of gout help them through the entire situation so that they do not have to face it alone. The more alone they feel, the more depressed and stressed out they will become. If they know that they have people around them who care for them and will be there for them especially when they suffer the most, they will be in a much happier state of mind.

Gout itself is quite a painful disease. When it is combined with factors such as depression, stress, and anxiety, it becomes intolerable. Therefore, a person should try and make sure that this point is not reached and they keep receiving the care that they need and require.

Conclusion

While gout is a significant disease, many people are not even aware of it. The majority of the people who have gout are completely clueless with regards to how the issue can lead to even greater concerns later on in life if proper measures are not taken. Therefore, proper education and awareness is important in this regard so that people can become more vigilant. This way, people who do not suffer from gout can take proper measures to avoid it later on in life and those who do can take steps to ensure that they take care of it and lead a healthy life despite having gout.

A very important thing to take into account is that people who do suffer from gout would benefit a lot if they have people around them to help them through the condition. It is a known fact that gout is painful, and with severe gout attacks, a person becomes bedridden and unable to move. They would require and appreciate an immense amount of help with reducing their pain and helping them get their daily chores done.

If the people who suffer from gout take proper measures to ease their pain they can lead much better and healthier lives. They will also suffer from less gout attacks and will be more comfortable overall.

This book has hopefully given you a detailed insight into gout and how you can best take care of the condition. Thank you for reading.

Published by IMB Publishing 2015

Made in the USA
Monee, IL
02 November 2019